*Aphrodisiacs*

# *Aphrodisiacs*
## *A Guide to What Really Works*

### Esmond Choueke

A Citadel Press Book
Published by Carol Publishing Group

Copyright © 1998 Esmond Choueke
All rights reserved. No part of this book may be reproduced in any form, except by a newspaper or magazine reviewer who wishes to quote brief passages in connection with a review.

A Citadel Press Book
Published by Carol Publishing Group
Citadel Press is a registered trademark of Carol Communications, Inc.

Editorial, sales and distribution, rights and permissions inquiries should be addressed to Carol Publishing Group, 120 Enterprise Avenue, Secaucus, N.J. 07094.

In Canada: Canadian Manda Group, One Atlantic Avenue, Suite 105, Toronto, Ontario M6K 3E7

Carol Publishing Group books may be purchased in bulk at special discounts for sales promotion, fundraising, or educational purposes. Special editions can be created to specifications. For details, contact Special Sales Department, Carol Publishing Group, 120 Enterprise Avenue, Secaucus, N.J. 07094.

Manufactured in the United States of America
10 9 8 7 6 5 4 3 2 1

Library of Congress Cataloging-in-Publication Data

Choueke, Esmond.
    Aphrodisiacs : a guide to what really works / Esmond Choueke.
      p. cm.
    ISBN 0-8065-1997-5 (pbk.)
    1. Aphrodisiacs.  I. Title.
RM386.C483  1998
615'.766—dc21
                                                       98–13659
                                                            CIP

*To love and making love*

# Contents

|  |  |
|---|---|
| Acknowledgments | ix |
| Important Note to Readers | xi |
| Introduction | xiii |

1. **The Joys of Aphrodisiacs** — 3
   - Analyzing Your Desires — 3
   - The Postage-Stamp Erection Test — 12
   - Choosing the Aphrodisiac That Will Work Best for You — 17

2. **Sharing Aphrodisiacs With Your Mate** — 35
   - Exercise — 36
   - Erotic Videos — 42
   - Music — 48
   - Location, Location, Location — 51
   - Miscellaneous Tricks — 58
   - Spiritual Aspects of Aphrodisiac Use — 60

3. **Herbal and Plant Aphrodisiacs** — 63
   - Yohimbine — 63

|   |   |   |
|---|---|---|
|    | Damiana | 70 |
|    | Avena Sativa | 72 |
|    | Muira Puama | 76 |
|    | Gingko Biloba | 79 |
|    | Dong Quai | 81 |
| 4. | *The New Pharmacological Substances* | 85 |
|    | The "Magic" Erection Pills | 85 |
|    | The Date-rape Pill | 94 |
|    | Erection Creams | 96 |
|    | Injection Therapy | 97 |
| 5. | *Modern Pharmaceuticals* | 101 |
|    | L-arginine | 102 |
|    | Niacin | 104 |
|    | Deprenyl | 105 |
|    | Bromocriptine | 108 |
| 6. | *The Aphrodisiac Feast* | 113 |
| 7. | *Miscellaneous Aphrodisiac Information* | 121 |
|    | Animal Products | 121 |
|    | Spanish Fly | 123 |
|    | Vacuum Devices and Penile Implants | 123 |
|    | Mixing and Matching | 124 |
|    | Selected Bibliography | 125 |

# *Acknowledgments*

I would like to thank those who took the time to share their aphrodisiac experiences with me on my e-mail site or on the live phone chat lines. For those who want to contribute their earthshaking, crazy, funny, yucky, steamy hot, or freezing cold sexual experiences to the upcoming sequel to this book, please post your message to **Aphrostory@aol.com**.

I would also like to thank Johan Santesson, webmaster of the Aphrodisiacs Exchange, for his advice and for sharing his vast files; William Glitz, media director of the American Urological Association, for putting me in touch with top U.S. urologists; and Hillel Black and Monica Harris, my editors at Carol Publishing.

*Important Note to Readers*

It is not the intention of the author or publisher to make any recommendations or accept responsibility for the use of any of the substances dicussed herein. Any such decisions should be made in consultation with a knowledgeable physician.

## Introduction

Taking aphrodisiacs effectively is as much an art as a science. To develop *Aphrodisiacs: A Guide to What Really Works,* I interviewed psychologists, urologists and other physicians, sex therapists, herbalists, and couples and singles just like you. I sifted through facts, myths, and *very* personal experiences to prepare this overall view of the best types of aphrodisiacs available. Some substances work better at different times, and some will work better for you than others—but success depends on delightful experimentation by you and your mate. The best way to maximize your sexual prowess and satisfaction through aphrodisiacs is to vary the types you use, just as you vary the sexual techniques and positions you use.

In earlier times, aphrodisiacs were sought out mainly by sultans and kings and other male leaders so that they could fornicate with as many "wives" as possible. Enterprising women used them secretly to ensnare unsuspecting men.

As we approach the year 2000, we see a new approach to using aphrodisiacs. They're now considered to be "recreational tools" that can be enjoyed by all ages and both genders whenever the urge to try something new in lovemaking strikes. Coast-to-coast sales of aphrodisiacs have soared into the hundreds of millions of dollars a year. This figure will double and triple as amazing new aphrodisiacs come on the market. These modern substances from the latest in medical science have succeeded in coming close to answering our ancestors' dreams for the perfect aphrodisiac.

With more aphrodisiacs to explore than ever, *Aphrodisiacs, A Guide to What Really Works*, will lead you down the path of orgasmic discovery. To choose what's best for you at any given time, listen to your beating heart and listen to the heartbeat of your mate.

*Aphrodisiacs*

# 1

# The Joys of Aphrodisiacs

### Analyzing Your Desires

A common theme has emerged from the experts interviewed for this book: In the 1990s, people are as much concerned about making their partner feel great during sex as they are about making themselves feel great.

"When patients ask me how they can enhance their sexual experiences through aphrodisiacs, they always ask if the substance will work equally well on their lovers," said Dr. Lyle Waldman, a Belgian-trained physician who prescribes aphrodisiacs to couples. "Men don't want to just get a hot erection and have a wonderful orgasm—they want their wives or girlfriends to be equally satisfied. As for women, in the past they'd seek out preparations solely to encourage erections in their husbands or boyfriends, but now they want to try the preparations at the same time so both can be equally pleased."

One couple interviewed for this book, Tracie and George, took their first aphrodisiac (a preparation featuring powdered damiana leaves) together, and expressed more delight in their partner's joys than their own. They had been married for eight years, had two sons, and were happy with their lives, but were looking for ways to spice up their love life.

Tracie said, "We took the damiana capsules together for a few days in a row before our eighth anniversary. We weren't expecting anything really, but I began to feel 'earthier' day by day, and started having more sexual fantasies than usual. On the fifth day, we came home from a cocktail party, sent the babysitter home, and turned out the lights while we snuggled on the living room couch. The damiana somehow made us feel more animalistic, and we began groping each other right there. We both felt really turned on. I realized that the lips of my vagina were tingly and warm, making me especially receptive to George. In fact, I was dying to feel his penis entering me—I wanted to suck him into me, like a vacuum cleaner, and hold his erection within me while I clutched him with my arms and legs. I wanted him to enjoy my own tingly vibrations and feel them as powerfully as I was, so that I could invigorate his whole being through his erection. I was sure the special feeling in my vagina would enter through his penis and spread to the rest of him, from his toes to his nose—and that he'd feel just as elated as I felt!

"When he did enter me, I had an even greater surprise," Tracie continued. He was already kind of vibrating from the effects of the damiana, and his vibrating cock and body turned me on even more. It seemed as if the more excited I became, the more excited he became, and vice versa. The damiana was making both of us feel earthy and lustful.

Neither of us wanted to climax because the buildup felt so wonderful on its own. But his thrusting and quivering took me over the limit, and I came in gushes of pleasure. A minute later, he too was overcome, and he was as overwhelmed as I was about the strength of his orgasm."

Tracie added, "We both realized that we had enabled one another to reach a peak experience—and we were both overjoyed by that. It made our bonds as a couple seem so much stronger and more tangible. I don't know if we ever felt more love between us than we did that evening."

George, who was listening in on Tracie's description of the grand event, said, "I got such a kick out of seeing Tracie go nuts when she came that I almost wouldn't have minded if I didn't come myself. Her face took on this amazing expression of pleasure and need—and I was the one who was bringing it on. Sometimes when I'm at the office I picture her expression of ecstacy in my mind, and it makes me feel turned on all over again. To me, that was the most fun of our first aphrodisiac experience—to see her get so excited."

This example shows that an important first step in selecting an aphrodisiac is to analyze your desires and expectations for sexual frequency, intensity, and orgasmic ecstacy. Like a lot of us, Tracie and George were having satisfactory sex, but it had become too predictable. Their orgasms were far from earth-shattering. The damiana experience made them feel different—in this case, "earthier"—and reignited the lust.

Other aphrodisiacs, such as the new chemicals we'll discuss later, are geared toward making a man achieve a firmer, stronger, and longer-lasting erection rather than toward making orgasms feel better. These chemicals can even make men who have been impotent for years feel as if they're

Masters of the Universe when they get their powerful erections! Still other aphrodisiacs have their main effect in increasing your desire for sex, while others make your sex organs more sensitive to stimulation.

After analyzing the substances outlined in this book, you'll be better able to decide which type of aphrodisiac will satisfy you and your mate at any particular point in time.

For instance, one aphrodisiac that is geared as much toward women as men is niacin, or Vitamin B-3. It acts rather quickly by inducing the production of histamine within the body, thus eliciting a copycat sexual flush—and many women say they have very intense orgasms when taking it.

Nancy, a thirty-four-year-old single woman who had multiorgasmic experiences while using hashish as a teenager, hoped to find a legal substance that would bring back those "flights to the moon." She turned to niacin, which did give her a mind-and-body "rush" similar to that produced by hash, and which also brought back her multiorgasmic experience.

"At a herbalist store, I read that niacin can give you something called a 'niacin flush'—sort of like a full-body blush," Nancy confessed. "It sounded good to me, so I thought I'd give it a try for my next sexual experience.

"I tried it the first time without a partner, just before taking a nice hot bath and going to bed. I wanted to see if I really would feel any effect, and I was very pleasantly surprised. My whole body took on an overall glow, and that included my mouth and genital area. I lay in my bed and played with my clitoris and vulva with my fingers, and it felt really, really good. In short order I had a lovely, pulsing orgasm."

She added, "I made up my mind to have niacin sex for the first time with a guy I had been dating. When we were out for drinks one night, I took a hundred-milligram capsule and invited my date to take one too. After all, it said 'Vitamin B-3' on the capsule, so it couldn't be too dangerous or weird. I invited him back to my apartment to listen to some CD's, and I think he was hoping to get lucky that night because he kept putting his arm around me and trying to be attentive as we walked home. I could have told him I was a sure bet, but I think it was more fun to keep him on edge."

Nancy, an engineer, continued, "By the time we reached my place, I was getting those hot, full-body blushes all over me, and I was simply horny as hell. It was all I could do to pretend that I was letting *him* seduce *me,* and soon enough we were both naked on my sheets. He was so happy at this encounter that he went down on me, but I was so hot down there that even his tongue felt rough on my clitoris. My mouth, though, was very sensitive, and I was dying to suck on his cock and feel it inside my mouth. The sensation of his erection on my 'blushing' lips and tongue was excellent. I made sure not to lick or suck too much because I wanted to experiment with having his penis inside my newly blushing vagina, and I didn't want him to just come inside my mouth. I put a condom on him, lay on my back, and guided his cock into me."

"The intercourse felt better than ever, even better than when I was on hash as a coed. I was so ready to come that I climaxed the first time within thirty seconds, and it felt like I was flying to the moon. I told him to go slow because I wanted him to last as long as possible, and I was released in orgasms three more times. It was wonderful. I became so wet down there I was a bit embarrassed! He came after a while, and that was fine with me, because I felt weak from coming so many times."

"We went out for a while, but it was a bit difficult dealing with him after that because the sex was so good for him too. He thought I must be in love with him since I came so many times....But I wasn't. He even sent me flowers and began trying to get serious. I didn't have the heart to tell him I was just using him to explore my sexuality, and I eventually let him down gently. I guess he still thinks he's Mister Stud! In any case, I'm ready to try another aphrodisiac or to use niacin again whenever I get another guy lined up," Nancy concluded.

Carl, a forty-nine-year-old man who dreamed of having "exquisite" sex with two women on the same weekend, confessed that he took yohimbine every day during a month to set himself up for the special occasion. Yohimbine, the inner bark of an African tree, has been used on that continent for centuries to boost the sexual response—and it worked for Carl for his recreational-sex weekend. In fact, many of the respondents who shared their experiences for this book cited "finding new kicks" as the main reason they indulged in the use of aphrodisiacs.

Carl, who lives in Miami, explained that he had been dating one woman steadily there when he met another woman on a business trip who openly flirted with him. She was going to visit Miami soon.

Said Carl, "Since I was a teenager, I had a dream of having sex with two women, one after the other, but I got married and it never happened. After my divorce, the idea still seemed really exciting, so when the opportunity came around, I planned to fulfill my fantasy like a military operation. I wanted to be a real he-man for both women. Frankly, I didn't question the moral implications of cheating on my girlfriend because we had an open relationship."

Carl added, "A herbalist I saw advised me to take yohimbine along with Siberian ginseng each day. He said the combination would work better and faster than either of the substances alone. Actually, about a week after starting the combination treatment, my girlfriend and I both noticed the difference. I was hornier and more orgasmic, and she gave me a lot of compliments about my sexual prowess. I kept on taking both pills each day so by the end of the month, I knew I'd be as strong as a bull.

"The day of reckoning finally arrived, and I spent Friday and Saturday night with my girlfriend as usual. We had sex each night, but my cock was still not satisfied. It almost had a mind of its own, wanting to find another available pussy. On Sunday afternoon, I met up with the other woman at her hotel. It was a hot day, so we swam and lay on deck chairs at the pool together. I was so hard and horny I couldn't walk around the pool without holding a towel in front of my erect cock! We took the elevator going up to her room, and I think she got the vibes off me about my urgent feelings. She began clinging to me right there, and we almost began having sex standing up in the elevator! In her room, we dropped onto the bed and began kissing and screwing and laughing about silly jokes. It was a great time. My penis was so hard and strong that it made the sex truly exquisite, just as I had dreamed it would be. The combination of the yohimbine and ginseng was working exactly as planned. We went out for dinner and then came back and screwed again. It was wonderful. My penis did feel pretty worn out by then, and I realized I wouldn't want to keep up that much sexual activity every weekend, but my sexual dream was fulfilled."

Carl concluded, "I've stopped taking the capsules and have resumed my normal sexual activity for now, but it's good to know that there are fun aphrodisiacs around which you can enjoy when you want to."

As previously noted, chemical aphrodisiacs are coming onto the market now that are far more powerful in inducing erections and sexual satisfaction than had previously been thought possible. Apart from benefiting people in fairly normal health, these new substances are a major breakthrough for men who have serious medical problems such as diabetes, prostate complications, hormone imbalance, high blood pressure, or partial paralysis. In these cases, the effects of the new chemicals in eliciting erections are truly startling.

Dr. Ira Sharlip, a San Francisco–based urologist who is a director of the Society for the Study of Impotence and a member of the American Urological Association, explained, "Urologists now have very effective methods available to provide rigidity of the penis, including new oral pills that are proving to be highly successful. There also are mini-injections into the penis called intracavernous injections, little pellets inserted up the tip of the penis, surgical implants, and vacuum devices.

"But everybody is excited about the oral pills. They're a very important development for men. And since they act as vasodilators, they may prove beneficial in increasing women's sexual satisfaction as well." Dr. Sharlip noted that several of these new pills are being approved by the U.S. Food and Drug Administration for popular use.

Thus, for men facing erectile dysfunction due to serious medical problems, the best type of lovemaking aids will probably be these new medications, which have been undergoing extensive testing in the United States, England, Europe, and other parts of the world for years. The three main pills currently available are composed of sildenafil, apomorphine, and phentolamine. In general, these drugs almost guarantee an erection lasting from sixty to ninety minutes.

The pills come on the heels of erectile drugs administered by an injection into the skin of the penis or in the form of a tiny pellet inserted into the tip of the penis. These forerunners of the erection pills do bring on strong, long-lasting erections, but they have several undesirable effects. Reportedly, they're cumbersome and a bit painful. They can also be irritating to the urethra. But worse than this, they may cause priapism—an erection that stays for hours and won't go away. It's a very painful condition that can cause permanent penile damage if an erection persists for more than four hours. Priapism requires emergency treatment by a doctor or radiologist, involving an injection of a local anesthetic or an arterial procedure to relieve the buildup of blood pressure inside the penis. Luckily, the new erection pills rarely if ever cause these problems.

The use of the new chemicals does bring up the debate as to whether erectile dysfunction is based on psychological or physical factors. Increasingly, urologists are saying that it's much more of a physical problem, which has its basis in circulation and blood pressure. Although it's possible to take specific tests to see if a patient's problem is vascular, those tests are expensive and time-consuming, involve the use of special ultrasound equipment, and are often more trouble than they're worth. The trend among urologists will likely be to simply prescribe one or another of the erection pills and see if it works, since there are virtually no serious side effects to the pills when used as prescribed. Either the man gets an erection or he doesn't. If the pill works—which it does on 80

> ## The Postage-stamp Erection Test
>
> If you're not getting an erection no matter what you try, here's a simple test you can do to see if you're physically okay. It's called the postage-stamp test, and it works on the basis of the fact that men ordinarily have several erections while sleeping at night without remembering that they happened. Thus, you end up mistakenly thinking your sword is permanently dented. But if you use the postage-stamp test, you'll be able to see if you do have erections at night, which is an indication that you're physically fine for sex—and that you can benefit from various aphrodisiacs.
>
> Here's how you do it: Take a row of three or four stamps that are still joined together. Lick-and-stick them around your penis while it's in a flaccid state, then go to sleep. In the morning, check to see if the stamps have torn apart. If so, you've had at least one erection, so you know you're physically capable of having one. If not, you should consult a urologist for more intensive treatment.

percent of eligible patients—great. If it doesn't, then doctors may try the vascular tests to look for other problems. For men who want to try a simple test to see if they have at least a baseline degree of erectile function—which can then be magnified through the use of the right aphrodisiac—there's the Postage-stamp Erection Test.

Dr. Sharlip also pointed out that there are new topical creams being tested that may also prove to be beneficial. One such cream contains nitroglycerin as the active ingredient for vasodilation. He added, "Any type of aphrodisiac that works to help produce an erection has a place in patient use. Even though the evidence for herbal products, for instance, is mainly anecdotal, they are also useful for many men and women."

These new pills, which we'll analyze in chapter 4, are already being seen as miracle drugs. As clinical testing is completed and they gain FDA approval, the market for them is expected to match that of the standard aphrodisiacs—that is, approaching $1 billion a year.

The new pills definitely helped Kathy and Paul, a couple in their forties, who were in distress before turning to these pills for help. They explained that their sex lives had declined to a very inadequate level after Paul began treatment for high blood pressure a year earlier. His medication had the effect of decreasing his ability to stay erect. Said Kathy, forty-eight, "It made me feel nervous whenever Paul and I started making love because he'd so often become limp soon after he was inside me. He'd feel bad because he thought he was letting me down, and then I had to build up his ego. I didn't care so much about the lack of penetration and orgasms—I just felt lousy because Paul did. It made us both so nervous that we almost stopped screwing entirely because of the possibility of disappointment. I'd end up giving him a combination of a blow job and hand job once in a while because that was the only way he'd stay hard until he came. Meanwhile, he'd stimulate my clitoris and G-spot manually to bring me to orgasm. That was fine, but when it's the only sexual release we had we both felt like we were missing something intimate. The worst part of it was that Paul felt like he was letting me down. But all that changed after he got a few of the erection pills (sildenafil) through a British connection—and they worked instantly.

"The first time Paul took the pill he got hard right away. We lay down naked in bed as usual, and I sucked on his penis and played with it as I always do with my hands. It was quite a pleasure because it was so stiff and erect. Paul was obviously getting a lot of pleasure from it himself as I could see from the look on his face and the twitches in his cock. He had lots of confidence in that erection, let me tell you! It was like when we were newlyweds all over again."

Kathy added, "His erection stayed hard as a sabre when he pushed it into my vagina. We were able to laugh and talk and not worry about it going down. Now we call it our 'love pill,' and we often build a whole night around it. We go out for dinner or to a club where we can dance, and I get to rub my thigh against his hard-on for fun while we're swaying to the music. All night we're anticipating the bedroom sex we'll soon be enjoying, and it makes our love session that much more exciting. I often have more than one orgasm because he maintains his erection for so long. It's made our marriage so much stronger. It's like a miracle pill."

Like the "natural" aphrodisiacs, the erection-inducing pills don't have to be taken forever. Patients use them a few times and are then often able to have unmedicated intercourse for a while because the machinery has been primed and is ready for action, so to speak.

In the future, it's likely that the traditional herbal aphrodisiacs and the erection pills will be taken in conjunction with each other—a joining of the old and the new. This way couples will be able to vary their sexual experiences without the risk of becoming habituated to one substance or another.

The new pills have a vasodilating effect on women as well—which can also be enhanced with traditional aphrodisiacs. Some delightful testing will have to be conducted to maximize both genders' desires.

Physicians point out that the desire for aphrodisiacs is by no means concentrated in older couples. Young wives and husbands inquire about aphrodisiacs almost as often as older couples do. One of the prime times they make this type of request is shortly after the couple has a new baby.

In one case, the newly popular capsules of St. John's Wort turned out to have an aphrodisiac effect.

Dr. Lyle Waldman, of Montreal, explained, "A patient named Debbie, twenty-nine, had two babies—a three-year-old and a one-year-old. She was concerned that her breasts didn't feel 'sexy' anymore to her. She used to love it when her husband caressed her, but no longer. She had already stopped breast-feeding for more than two months and was expecting her previous erotic feelings to return—but they didn't.

"Debbie told me, 'Before, when my husband would play with my nipples, it made me really excited—but now, nothing.' It was clear that she was pretty run down from taking care of the kids, and she seemed mildly depressed—so I prescribed a course of St. John's Wort. Even though it's not officially an aphrodisiac, it had that type of effect on her because it relieved her anxiety and the mild depression caused by the stress of taking care of two little babies. That helped make her body feel more sensual to her.

"Just a month later, Debbie told me that she was feeling more optimistic and happier overall, and that she was enjoying sex again. That mild herbal boost provided just the right kind of help she needed to get her sexual response back to her normal level. Importantly, St. John's Wort doesn't have the anti-orgasmic effects of other popular antidepressants."

Dr. Waldman added, "If the situation arises that a husband is the one who's nervous that he's lost interest in sex, I prescribe yohimbine, which is an item the FDA has approved for this use. Usually, the husband will notice beneficial results within a couple of weeks."

One of the questions Dr. Waldman's patients ask him is whether an aphrodisiac can change a person's sexual orientation. "That's a pretty funny question," he said. "If an aphrodisiac does make you hornier, it will only make you hornier for the object or objects of your desires. It's not as if an aphrodisiac will make you want to have intercourse with the first thing that comes along. That is, gays will seek out their own gender to vent their new lust on, and straights will want to have more sex with the opposite sex. If an aphrodisiac could have an effect on orientation, people would have been switching back and forth for centuries!"

If a woman is physically disabled in a way that prevents sexual satisfaction, physicians usually have the means to help her try to become orgasmic. For instance, a woman from a Third World country who had a clitorectomy as a young girl may find help in reaching orgasm with modern and traditional aphrodisiacs. Said Dr. Waldman, "If, for instance, the woman has lost her clitoris but still retains her vulva, she can increase the erotic sensations she feels on both the outside and inside of her vagina. Perhaps we'd start by prescribing niacin along with L-arginine (a natural amino acid) along with a lubricating cream that might contain estrogen. The goal would be to help her experience as much pleasureful sensation in and around her vagina as possible even though her clitoris had been removed. If both her vulva and clitoris are gone, she may be fortunate enough to have a G-spot that responds well. Some experimentation with various combinations of substances should yield orgasms."

These cases illustrate the point that people have different sexual cravings and different reasons for wanting to take an aphrodisiac—and that timing, physiology, and mental desire have an important influence on determining the most suitable substances. Experts note that aphrodisiacs can be seen either as a luxury or a necessity depending on your desires and needs.

### Choosing the Aphrodisiac That Will Work Best for You

Anyone who's perused the books and the research data concerning aphrodisiacs in his local library, bookstore, or Internet search engine can attest to the hundreds of different herbs, chemicals, animal products, and other preparations available. Some manufacturers hype their products so much you know they can't possibly live up to the ecstatic claims. Others come with testimonials from real people and medical details that make them seem genuine and worthy. Here, we'll sift through many of these claims and substances in order to provide a usable guide to what you and your partner should be trying and when.

In a broad sense, we can divide the available aphrodisiacs into four main categories that we'll analyze further: traditional herbal and plant preparations, erectile pills, other new pharmacological substances, and animal-based products. Regarding these animal-based products, there's a strong indication that most don't live up to their expansive claims involving sexual stimulation.

It's best for couples to discuss their particular desires and predicaments openly with each other and with their aphrodisiac supplier, be it a herbalist, homeopath, psychologist, or physician. Couples can then make an intelligent choice as to which aphrodisiac is best suited for them at a particular time in their lives.

Invariably, though, you shouldn't use the same aphrodisiac all the time. For one thing, you'll build up a tolerance for that substance and require more and more of it to have an effect. Second, experimentation is important so that you can try the different effects of different products for yourself. If you're a man, you may sometimes want a substance that gives you a firmer and bigger erection—but if it also tends to make you climax too soon, you may want to try something different. If you're a woman, you may be happiest with an aphrodisiac that elicits a fast orgasm compared to another that yields overall body sensitivity. The program that works best for most people is to begin a schedule of using one type of aphrodisiac for a few days or weeks, and then take a break for several weeks before trying another.

One common myth is that a person may become dependent on the use of aphrodisiacs, diminishing his or her natural sexual responses. As long as you change aphrodisiacs and give yourself a rest period, however, the opposite is true for most people. Yolande, who's in her fifties noted, "We had some wonderful sexual experiences when my husband and I started trying aphrodisiacs, but I was nervous that he wouldn't be able to get it up once he stopped taking the substances. I mean, after we experienced the gratifying orgasms and longer times for intercourse, would it mean that nonenhanced sex would become a nonevent? In the end, I had nothing to worry about. I found that taking the aphrodisiacs kick-started our love life from time to time. During the times when we were off them completely, we still had excellent sexual experiences in all forms—vaginal, oral, and manual. The aphrodisiacs are a way to feel sex differently. The aphrodisiacs help us maintain our interest and curiosity in our sexual response."

Many people report that this is also true for them. They'll try an aphrodisiac alone or in combination with other substances, evaluate the effects, see if they enjoy the experience, and then try a different combination a month later.

Regarding combinations, you'll find when choosing an aphrodisiac that virtually every substance can be bought either alone or in various mixtures. Often, a herbalist or homeopath will advise you to make a mixture yourself or will tell you to take two or three capsules of different items at the same time. One of the most common additives recommended is Siberian ginseng, which seems to give most aphrodisiacs a strong boost.

Charlie, sixty-three, found this combination to be beneficial when he tried damiana, the dried leaves of a shrub grown in hot climates. On their own, the green capsules didn't have any noticeable effect in the short run. But his wife suggested he take ginseng along with the damiana, and it had a surprising effect. He said, "I had lost interest in sex, and anyways I'm always too tired at night to do anything but fall asleep. But with these capsules I began getting spontaneous erections just as I used to get in high school. My wife noticed the difference right away. Now she often suggests that we have an 'afternoon delight' when she notices my cock is hard.

"Some afternoons she makes me drive her home quickly from the supermarket or wherever we are. She plays with my hard-on in the car because she thinks it's so 'cute'! We usually get right down to it when we get home. We just pull our clothes off and begin having intercourse on the sofa or floor. She says 'you have to shoot while the ducks are flying.' I think that's kind of true. She likes it as much as I do. Her vagina feels really tight these days, maybe because my boner gets so big. Luckily we both exercise every day, because our hearts wouldn't be able to keep up with so much sex activity if we weren't in good shape—we'd probably die of heart attacks! Can you believe it, at our age, we're carrying on like we did when we were first dating."

Another popular additive is alcohol in moderate amounts. One of the best ways of taking damiana is to marinate an ounce of the leaves in tequila for a week, and then mix a few tablespoons into a cup of tea. Many people south of the border swear that this is the best way of reaching sexual ecstasy—and claim that it produces a marijuana-like high.

Brazilians swear to the delights of a concoction they make from the bark and roots of the *muira puama* bush, the local counterpart of the African-based yohimbine tree. Both have been esteemed by natives for use in ritual gatherings for centuries. Modern Brazilians steep several tablespoons of crushed muira puama in half a pint of boiling vodka for fifteen minutes, then strain it and drink the mixture at their famous all-night dance parties. Said Angelina, who moved to the United States from Bahia, "Man, we sip that muira puama while we're dancing, and we just stay horny and excited all night. We keep on dancing for hours—and sometimes that seems more fun than sex. But before long you take a liking to some guy, and he dances near you, and you look at each other. The parties come to an end when the sun starts to come up, and everyone's totally drained of energy and dripping with sweat. That's when you take your guy and fall into someone's bed and have sex and more sex, and then sleep till noon, and fuck again."

Sarge, a fifty-five-year-old resident of the Four Corners area, noted that he uses vodka as an additive to wash down the dried snake skin powder he recommends as a sex enhancer. "It makes my cock feel nasty and strong. It makes me fuck fast and hard," he said.

In the East, expensive brands of cognac are mixed with such substances as snake bile, snake blood, and bat blood. While most Westerners cringe at the thought of swallowing things like live snake blood or bile (they bring the reptiles to the table and bleed them into a goblet in front of your eyes), in Asia they accept it as a matter of course. Said one man from Hong Kong, "Along with making your sperm very strong, snake bile also wards off colds for the entire winter, so why wouldn't everyone want to drink it?"

Many animal-based products commonly ingested in the East aren't well accepted in the Western world. Actually, the medical evidence to back up claims that animal-based products are good aphrodisiacs is far less positive than the evidence available regarding herbs and plants. For instance, although rhinoceros horn may sell for as much as $25,000 per pound in Asia, medical analysts say it's made of nothing more than keratin—the same type of tissue we find in our own hair and nails. If there is any active aphrodisiac ingredient, it's probably trace amounts of L-arginine, which can easily be bought in health food stores for just a few dollars per ounce. As long as the species of animal involved isn't endangered, however, and as long as you can be assured that no animals suffered in procuring these products, animal-based aphrodisiacs are something you may choose to try.

If the thought of ingesting this type of animal product makes you cringe, psychologists such as Dr. David Turkat of Atlanta Psychological Associates advise leaving them alone. "If you get a nauseous feeling in your gut at the mere thought of taking a product, it can easily prove to be a real turnoff during sex. But there's no harm in trying them."

One aphrodisiac, made of powdered sea horse skeletons, has proven so popular that the aqua-farming of sea horses has been developed into a profitable business in the Far East.

Usually, the most palatable way to ingest animal-based products is by taking them in their dried, powdered, encapsuled form. For instance, a common preparation from Chinese and Korean homeopaths and herbalists involves capsules containing several types of dried penis (such as seal, otter, and deer) along with powdered antlers. You can also buy whole, dried versions of these products—including items such as gallbladders and gallstones—and make a tea of them by shaving bits into a teapot with boiling water.

Perhaps a more palatable animal-based aphrodisiac is made from processed ambergris, a waxlike substance that floats on ocean waves and that is secreted from the intestines of sperm whales. This odiferous substance is found in tropical seas and is scooped up by commercial fishermen, usually near a shoreline or on beaches. It's sold to drug firms and herbalists who process it with various edible ingredients and turn it into a type of strong-tasting jujube candy or into an edible powder. During the French Renaissance, a touch of natural ambergris was simply smeared onto chocolates and eaten in anticipation of sexual encounters. The waxy substance is also mixed with flowery-smelling potions for use in perfumes and sensual massage ointments.

Joan, a forty-two-year-old divorcée from Oregon, notes

that her lover massaged her with an ambergris-based ointment they bought in Europe, and she found the feel and smell of it so intriguing and luxurious that she wanted to try it also in its edible form. She noted, "Ken told me that the ointment smelled a bit like a flowery cunt, and I thought he was kind of right. It was very pleasant, really. We went to the next stage in which we purchased and swallowed the prepared jellylike capsules of ambergris together, and it worked right away."

Joan continued, "We became totally horny, wanting to simply fuck each other. It wasn't even like making love. We just wanted to put our genitals together the moment after we took the capsules. We were watching a video in his rec room, and we found our hands groping each other's bodies—and then caressing each other's crotches. I began squeezing his penis. It had become really hard as a rock. Meanwhile, he was massaging my vagina with the palm of his hand under my skirt. It made me feel crazy—I wanted to rub my vagina all over his cock. I hiked up my skirt, yanked off my panties while he pulled off his trousers, and then I straddled him. His penis was so hard and eager that I was able to hold on to it tight with my hands and rub it over my clitoris again and again until I had a wonderful orgasm. Then I moved his cock so that it entered right into me, and by then he was pretty ready to come himself. His whole body twitched as he had his orgasm inside me, and I don't think I've ever gotten so full up with come in my life!"

The choice of aphrodisiacs is important for another reason—different ones work through different physical and mental mechanisms. We have already noted how some aphrodisiacs lead directly to greater genital arousal. For instance, niacin creates a physical sensation similar to blushing in the genitals; yohimbine leads to stronger erections, and damiana creates a tingling anticipation in the vulva, penis, and testicles. These three aphrodisiacs are considered to be mainly physically mediated.

Other aphrodisiacs start out as psychologically mediated, and then turn you on physically. That is, they increase the sexual response in women and men through brain-related processes.

For instance, an aphrodisiac in this category is L-arginine. It functions through a process that starts within the brain and then branches out to the sex organs. This substance works by increasing the production of the neuroactive chemical nitric oxide, or NO, which in turn leads to heightened sexual response in both men and women. In men, erections are created because the NO facilitates greater blood flow to the penis through the dilation of penile blood vessels, resulting in harder, bigger, and longer-lasting erections. Women also experience heightened sexual response due to the dilation of blood vessels of the vagina. There's also a bonus for men, since L-arginine often improves male fertility by increasing sperm motility.

Dr. Ellis Gottesfeld, an assistant professor at New York University's Department of Medicine, explained "Nitric oxide has emerged as a universally important molecule in terms of blood flow throughout the body. It has been known that it was important for erections, but it's also critical for blood flow to the heart and throughout the body. Essentially, it can be considered an aphrodisiac that starts in the brain and then affects the entire person."

A second neuroactive molecule whose production is increased through the use of L-arginine supplements is the hormone called GH or growth hormone. GH is almost a type of youth serum. In small doses, it can revitalize body tissues and increase the libido—making both men and women *feel* younger and hornier.

Thus, the question arises as to which type of aphrodisiac makes sex better for you and your mate—the psychologically mediated kind or the physically mediated kind. Once again, both are probably excellent at different times and for short periods. It's up to you and your mate to gain an understanding of the types of aphrodisiacs available and to evaluate which ones enhance your sex life the most.

Margaret, a thirty-four-year-old lawyer in New York, tried both types and noted that each has its benefits. She was most surprised after taking L-arginine supplements because she became multiorgasmic for the first time in her life, and she lauded their effectiveness. "Sex was always fun on its own. You know, I'd have an orgasm about two out of three times I had intercourse. And on the occasional time when I'd have a really energetic lover who went down on me or who did a lot of manual stimulation while his cock was inside me, I might come twice in one lovemaking session. With L-arginine, my pussy remains aroused even after having an orgasm—so it's pretty easy to have the second one. And both of them are very intense. My whole body feels like it's pulsating."

Margaret added, "I figured the sex would get even better if I could get my boyfriend to try it at the same time I did so that he'd be hornier as well. So I gave some to Garry, whom I'd been dating on and off for the past year, and he also became much hornier than usual. The first time we had arginine sex his cock stayed hard for a whole hour inside me. He said he loved the sensation of fucking me for so long (and the word 'love' is a word he doesn't use very often), and it seemed as if he was having a series of mini-comes until he finally ejaculated in big bursts. I came powerfully three times, and I walked around with a smile for a whole week. I could barely concentrate on my cases.

"We were so keen on the L-arginine supplements that he and I took them repeatedly for a month. But the thrill was gone eventually. I don't know if I lost interest in Garry or if the stuff just lost its effectiveness. We went back to unenhanced sex for a while, and things were back to normal—that is, good, but no cigar.

"Then I talked to a herbalist who advised trying another substance, a preparation of muira puama, steeped in alcohol—and it got us in the genitals right away. It was pretty funny, because one of the biggest differences between the two aphrodisiacs was how hot my pussy and Garry's cock became on this concoction. I swear, we could have boiled water by holding it on our genitals! We had fewer orgasms than with L-arginine, but the sex was fast, furious, and intense compared to the slower, more drawn-out screwing we did on L-arginine. Both items, though, get two thumbs up.

"It was fun trying both of those different types of sexual highs. Since then I've split up with Garry, and I plan on trying something different with my next boyfriend—whoever that turns out to be."

A couple in their sixties reported that L-arginine helped them feel better about their sexual activity. Bob said, "We both felt more energetic in our lovemaking, like it was more of a fun exercise to do instead of just plain having intercourse. It put us into a better *mood* while having sex, so it was a happy event. And we didn't tire out even after reaching orgasm. My wife and I went for walks after having sex on the L-arginine supplements, and we had a great time walking around and holding hands and feeling, well, *young* again."

These couples found satisfaction through brain-mediated aphrodisiacs but there was an unhappy couple as well. Sheila, forty-seven, and Sam, fifty, are a married couple in Canada who complained because Sam became too aggressive after taking the L-arginine supplement. Said Sheila, "I've read about what happens to athletes when they take steroids for too long, and I think the L-arginine supplements ended up having that effect on Sam. He thought it was fun to try rough sex with me after taking the supplements for a couple of weeks. He began by pulling my hair tight almost to the point of pain while ordering me to suck his cock. I didn't think that was very cool. He'd act as if he didn't know his own strength. And he'd bite my collarbone and hips, and then dig his nails into my buttocks really hard when he came. I mean, I was glad that he was having such intense sexual feelings, but it turned me off the more aggressive he became.

"I was used to Sam making love with me as if he really cared, even though I'd only come once in a while. I guess the first couple of times we had more aggressive sex while we were taking L-arginine I enjoyed his wrestling-type attack on me, but he took that as a license to get rougher. I felt that he didn't really care which woman he had between his legs—all he wanted was a vagina to shove his cock into as hard as possible and a womanly physique to vent his aggression on. I literally was just getting fucked, and I didn't enjoy the pain. I couldn't care less about the fact that I was probably more orgasmic. I finally told him it was the end of the L-arginine experiment for us—and he couldn't figure out what I was complaining about. I refused to have sex with him until the effects wore off a week later."

Sheila explained that the couple then turned to the milder forms of aphrodisiac herbs along with sensual massage. "I mentioned my rough experience on L-arginine to a dietician friend, and she suggested I try preparing some recipes that encourage lovemaking instead of taking a real aphrodisiac. She explained that some of the foods that are traditionally thought of as having aphrodisiac qualities do contain important supplements. For instance, oysters contain high levels of zinc and other minerals. Well, we've eaten oysters before with no sexual results. This time around, we took some yohimbine before going to a seafood restaurant, and I told Sam in advance that we'd probably start screwing like crazy again if we ate oysters—and I think the suggestion made him very horny and happy indeed. And that was sexy enough for me."

The imbalance between Sheila and Sam in terms of sexual harmony brings to light another important choice to make—are there times when only one partner should take an aphrodisiac? The answer is yes. In a situation where one partner is experiencing a decrease in sexual desire while the other remains as libidinous as ever, it would be prudent for only the partner experiencing the decreased libido to take the aphrodisiac. This way, the less interested partner will rise to the same level as his or her mate, equaling the lovers' sexual energy. If both partners in this situation take an aphrodisiac, the hornier one would just become more so and the other would never catch up.

"Nobody likes being pestered into having sex when they're not interested. So I'd advise people who want to increase their libido to make sure their partners will be happy about it," Dr. Turkat said.

A woman named Alicia, fifty-five, had a sad tale concerning this type of dilemma. After thirty years of marriage, her husband seemed to have lost interest in her, and they rarely had sex. She thought she'd surprise him by buying an aphrodisiac they could take together, and she brought home a preparation containing damiana and muira puama. He reluctantly agreed to take it with her for a few days, and he did begin having sex with her occasionally. Unfortunately, she was the one who became tremendously aroused—and ended up being more frustrated than ever. "My own desire for sex went up, and I was surprised about how good it could feel after many years of so-so sex. Although Bill did it with me a bit more than usual, he couldn't come close to matching my new arousal level. I became resentful that he didn't seem to care anymore, so I let myself be seduced by one of the widowers in the bridge league. At my age I felt I had nothing to lose—besides, it was fun to be wild for once in my life. Well, that widower bragged to one of his pals, who told my husband, and now we're getting divorced. It wasn't worth it. I should have taken something to decrease my desire, or I should have just given something to Bill and not taken anything at all myself."

Timing is also important for couples taking aphrodisiacs. Lewis, a fifty-three-year-old oil rig worker who was away from his wife for three months, said, "I hadn't had any sex at all while I was at the rig site, and what happened to me was that I completely forgot about sex. Being in a gang of men like that and working until you're exhausted every day totally saps your sex drive. About a week before I was going back home one of the guys sold me a bottle of an African aphrodisiac that had avena sativa (an extract of wild green oats) and yohimbine in it, and he told me the loving would be twice as good if I took it. So I took a couple of capsules a day for a week before flying back—and when I got there my wife announced she had to fly to her mother's because she was sick. We hardly had time to have sex even once before she was gone—and there I was for days, getting hard-ons all the time. I ended up having to masturbate to make my cock go down."

Finally, regarding currently available pharmacological drugs, there has been much discussion about chemicals that were developed for use in the treatment of Parkinson's and Alzheimer's—but that also act as strong aphrodisiacs. Many women and men are now experimenting with these drugs to boost their sexual prowess even though they don't have any cognitive problems.

Dr. Dan Shalom, a San Francisco–based neurologist, explained, "Substances such as deprenyl, bromocriptine, and L-dopamine often reawaken a latent sexual drive. In a clinical setting, these drugs are usually given to patients in their sixties. They're usually effective for several years for the treatment of these neurological diseases.

"The unexpected bonus discovered by many patients was that they were able to resume having sexual relations even after being unable to do so for years, thanks to these drugs."

The newest of these three drugs is deprenyl, a substance recently introduced to the United States by a Canadian-based company that imported it from Europe, where it has been used widely for more than a decade. Deprenyl greatly decreases tremors in Parkinson's patients, many of whom called the drug "miraculous" in its ability to help them lead normal lives. Deprenyl was also found to have a rejuvenating and aphrodisiac effect in both humans and animals.

An insider working with deprenyl noted, "It was an open secret among those who tried deprenyl in the beginning that it really drove up the sex lives of the men who were taking it. But it couldn't be promoted that way because it could lead to adverse reactions from the FDA."

Recently, people without neurological problems have been able to get prescriptions for deprenyl and other drugs in this category from physicians for aphrodisiac purposes, through so-called "off-label" prescriptions. (This is a legal method of obtaining a drug for a use outside of that stated on the label.)

One seventy-one-year-old man with Parkinson's who started a course of deprenyl reported with great pleasure that he began waking up with a hard-on every morning just as he did when he was young. Said Ivan, "My wife had passed away about five years earlier, and I hardly had any sexual experiences at all since then. Frankly, I had lost interest in sex, especially after my Parkinson's tremors began a year ago.

"When I read about deprenyl, I immediately asked my doctor to prescribe it, and I was totally pleased that my tremors decreased to almost nil after a few days. That was the first miracle. Then came the second: my boners! I began with the morning boner, and then I'd get spontaneous erections during the day. It was so funny at my age. My penis felt like my old pal again.

"On the same floor of my apartment building was a young and warm thirty-four-year old woman whom I'd often exchange pleasantries with. I'm sure she never thought of me in a sexual way, and I never thought about sex anymore anyway, so that didn't crop up—until my new boners began appearing. Once in a while, when I used to bump into her, I'd ask her over for coffee, but after getting my newfound bursts of libido, I began asking her over for a cocktail or to watch a late-night movie. I was surprised by my own audacity. I think the deprenyl gave me the urge, the energy, and the positive outlook. In fact, I think some of my new feelings must have rubbed off on her.

"Before I knew it, that woman, Sophie, began inviting me over to her place too. I certainly began to feel romantic and turned on by her, and she started feeling something too. I know she was even more surprised than I was at the thought of having sexual urges toward an old goat like me. But I was an energetic old goat who was a lot of fun with my newly-erectable 'toy.' And my physique is pretty good. That's because the tremors I used to have in my muscles improved their strength and definition. Finally, we went up to the exercise room in our building one night, and we got into the hot whirlpool together. Our bodies were pretty close together, and my arm went around her.

"Sophie snuggled right up to me in her bikini. Her bare skin against me drove me wild. I hadn't been that excited for many years! She could obviously feel the hard bulge in my bathing suit, and she squeezed it firmly in her hands. She looked amazed. She turned around to face me and began pressing into me. I knew young girls are more aggressive than in my day, but I didn't know they were *that* aggressive."

Ivan continued, "Sophie pulled the crotch of her bikini to the side, and slid my bathing suit down toward my knees, so that my boner was totally exposed beneath the swirling hot water—and then she rubbed my cock against her vagina until it opened up for me like a flower. And we started having intercourse right there. We didn't kiss much, but the connection between my cock and her vagina was like fireworks.

"For months after, Sophie would pop in from time to time to my place for a quickie. It was great."

Ivan added, "The effects of the deprenyl have been very positive for more than a year so far. But my affair with Sally ended soon after anyway. I guess I'll see what the future holds for me. But it sure was great having that experience—it was like being reborn."

Another prescription drug, bromocriptine, used for both Parkinson's and Alzheimer's, is being tried with success by people who want to boost their sexual activity. Donald, forty-one, reported that he was "knocked to the floor" by the sensational orgasms he experienced while taking it. He provided some evidence to support the theory that bromocriptine can lead to super-high levels of sexual excitement or hypersexuality. "I had at least six orgasms in a row, and they felt like they had the power of a piledriver in overdrive. I just couldn't stop making myself have orgasms when I was screwing my girlfriend—it was almost like eating potato chips," Donald said.

Bromocriptine is also reported to have a libido-enhancing effect on women, especially postmenopausal women. (One important warning is that this drug can restart ovulation in postmenopausal women, and may bring about an unwanted pregnancy.)

Lucy, sixty-three, explained that she had lost interest in sex and participated in occasional intercourse with her husband only to please him. She hadn't experienced an orgasm in more than a year. Two weeks after taking her prescription for bromocriptine, however, she became "normally" arousable again. "One night it seemed as if my clitoris and vagina had emerged from a shell and were anxious to feel the pleasures of sex again. That evening I urged my husband to come to bed early, and he was pretty surprised when I began massaging his penis. He was used to my just lying back with my knees up waiting for him to do his thing to me. But I really was enjoying it when he put his penis in me this time, and I couldn't stop myself from groaning with pleasure. That made him very pleased with himself! I didn't have an orgasm that night, but I did a few days later, and pretty much all the time after that. It made me feel like a young woman again, and it made me believe in aphrodisiacs"

These drugs have few harmful side effects as long as the products are taken as directed. Usually the side effects, if any, are listed clearly on the bottles. The most common can be rapid heartbeat or digestive irregularities. As for all such products, if you're in doubt or if you have any unusual medical problem, you should discuss the matter with your doctor.

For the aphrodisiacs described in this chapter, possible undesirable side effects usually result from overdosing or from being particularly sensitive. Be alert for these: Niacin may irritate ulcers; damiana and yohimbine in giant doses may cause stomach upset; L-arginine can raise blood sugar levels and shouldn't be taken by diabetics; L-arginine can also lengthen the time it takes to heal from a herpes attack; bromocriptine and deprenyl may cause temporary stomach upset, headache, and changes to blood pressure.

As for the plant and animal preparations custom-made by herbalists and homeopaths, there haven't been many reported medical problems, but each concoction is different and users should make note of what they're taking.

# 2

# *Sharing Aphrodisiacs With Your Mate*

It's great to mix aphrodisiacs with the whole range of activities that turn you and your mate on, according to many couples and health professionals. In general, the activities end up making the aphrodisiac's sexual stimulation even more pronounced, as you can see from the examples below. This should give you an idea of the range of possibilities to explore while trying your favorite substances, so that you can go on to your own discoveries.

An important note comes from psychologist Dr. Turkat of Atlanta. He explained that turning on your loved one involves a mix of caring about what he or she likes and sharing what you like. "In aspects of sex and relationships, you usually obtain the highest satisfaction by taking care of your mate's needs along with your own. If you stick with this concept, you'll be able to encourage each other on to greater emotional and sexual highs. And if either or both of you enjoy using aphrodisiacs, you can introduce them into your routine."

"It's good to explore and act on each other's desires and fantasies as long as the two of you are in agreement. Why should sex become boring for either partner? It must have been exciting when the two of you first met, so it's important to make the effort to keep your sexual relationship stimulating and exciting as time goes by."

## *Exercise*

One of the biggest and oldest myths about encouraging sexual activity involved the idea that to get turned on, both partners should be lounging around in a state of total relaxation. This concept seems to have been handed down from the ancient Romans and Greeks, in images of them lying on their backs as they dangled bunches of grapes above each other's mouths. But we see now that it's really an active life which promotes better sex.

A recent study by the Human Sexual Psychophysiology Lab at the University of Washington showed convincingly that exercise boosts the libido—especially in women. The report noted that a woman's sexual arousal is increased when her heartbeat and breathing rate rise while exercising. For instance, the researchers show that riding an exercise bike for half an hour makes women feel hornier than doing something ostensibly romantic, like having a candlelight dinner.

Dr. Waldman from Montreal said, "Taking aphrodisiacs before or during exercise can greatly increase their power. That's because your metabolism speeds up, and more of the active compounds can be used by the body. Like many other substances, aphrodisiacs will have a more intense effect on you if your cardiovascular system is pumped up. For instance, if you've already tried yohimbine, try it again before a workout, and see how much more sexually aroused you become.

"Exercise in itself is great as a prelude to sex. Think about it: You're breathing hard, your heart is pumping inside your chest, beads of sweat are forming all over your body, and you experience a deep heat from within. Your genitals feel as pumped up as the rest of you. It can lead to some pretty intense sexual activity and orgasms, especially after adding an aphrodisiac into the equation. That's one of the tips I give my patients who want to improve or restart their sex lives."

Dr. Waldman added, "I also point out that you should become more fit overall and quit smoking if you are smoking. Sex involves the whole body, especially the cardiovascular system, so being in good shape is a good first step. Sex involves a lot of exertion and a fair amount of calisthenic-type activity. If you're not up to it, you may be missing out on great orgasms. For instance, you can find yourself in a controlling position sexually with your mate between your legs, and you sense an orgasm is imminent. Yet you end up being too tired to move your hips and body as energetically as you'd like to. You get all tired out, and you end up missing the climax. Or you may never actually get close to climaxing simply because you're too fatigued.

"In general, you should do the amount of exercise that's comfortable for you, sticking to the general formula of boosting your heart rate by 30 percent for 30 minutes or more, four times a week." You may find that your aphrodisiac's strength has increased greatly because of the improvement in your blood flow during exercise, so you should be careful not to take too high a dose.

"To sum it all up, being in good shape makes you and your mate respond better sexually, and adding an aphrodisiac into the equation will make its libido-enhancing effects even greater," Dr. Waldman concluded.

Many of those who discussed their experiences for this book confirmed that their favorite aphrodisiac substances worked better than ever when they were more physically active.

Letitia, forty-eight, wrote, "My husband and I have more sex and better sex now than when we were married twenty years ago—and that's because we don't hang around for Happy Hour in bars boozing up after work like we used to. Instead we work out or go for a swim, and we both feel energized. Sometimes we massage each other with a pheromone-laced cream after exercising, or, if we're feeling really wild, we take a capsule of niacin.

"Niacin really gives you a whammo feeling after exercise. There's a whole-body flush that's really pronounced, and my vagina feels like it's got a built-in vibrator humming away. Our routine starts in our den where we have a treadmill and stationary bike. My husband Ross, who's forty-five, and I take turns on the machines for about twenty minutes each while watching the TV news. Even without an aphrodisiac, my vagina feels really *ready* for sex after that workout—but if I take niacin in between the treadmill and bike, it turns me into a red-hot volcano of sexual lust at the end of my workout. I'm almost at the point of desperation to get laid. My husband is usually pumped up by then too, and I'm so ready for him that our orgasms bring on a deep sexual rush that shakes both of our bodies entirely. The niacin experience is really very intense—and is *not* for everyday use!"

Letitia added, "On occasion, Ross is in the mood to take one of the capsules as well, and he gets a kick out of it because his penis becomes ten times more sensitive and his orgasm has a great *whoosh* to it, or so he says. But the intensity seems to make him come faster. I prefer screwing for a longer period of time, so when he does take the niacin I have him masturbate me during foreplay and that makes me come before he penetrates me."

"To me, exercise plus a sexual stimulant is the perfect combination."

A tennis-playing couple in New Jersey, Caroline and Richard, both thirty-four, decided to get engaged after they got hooked on their post-tennis arginine-and-ginseng sex sessions. Richard said, "When Caroline and I started dating each other seriously, we had nice, warm sex and it was excellent. For an adventure, a friend of mine suggested I try an aphrodisiac from an herbalist in New York, and I convinced Caroline that it should be fun. The preparation he gave us mainly had yohimbine and ginseng in it, and he gave me zinc pills to take at the same time because zinc is supposed to make an orgasm more wild. It was quite an exciting addition to our lovemaking. We'd get a new high-energy glow between us after we took the capsules. Our physical contacts were really exciting, even when we were just holding and touching each other, especially when we'd be naked. It was luxurious to feel her rubbing her breasts all over my chest and feel her fingers massaging me all over my body. Sex was just the icing on the cake after those warm, romantic feelings.

"It all became even better when Caroline suggested

taking the capsules in the afternoon before we went out to play tennis. The effect was unbelievable. After whacking the ball over the net for an hour and getting really hot and sweaty, that 'glowing' feeling I usually get grew into a steaming funk. *I was hot for her—no two ways about it!* She was also very turned on, and we kept caressing each other as we walked off the courts. There was no way I'd have been able to get into our club's swimming pool—everyone would have laughed their heads off at the stiff rod in my bathing suit! We were barely able to make it back to our apartment before our passion overwhelmed us and we tore off each other's clothes. It was very endearing how we began making love while hugging each other as tightly as those little stuffed monkeys you buy at amusement parks. It sounds corny, but it made us feel like one person rather than two separate people.

"Afterward, we just lay around for an hour with the sun shining through the window, talking about little things that made us laugh and cry. The aphrodisiac-enhanced love was a total experience. The feelings we shared formed one extra loop in the chain that convinced us that we were right for each other. I mean, if she enjoys that amount of closeness as much as I do, and if she's even willing to be as adventurous as I am, it means there's so much we can share together. After that summer of tennis and love, I asked her to marry me. She said okay (I think because to her it was another adventure!), and we've been happy ever since."

One other type of exercise that lends itself to aphrodisiac use is bowling, according to Geraldine, sixty-six. "A lot of us widows and divorcées get together on Wednesday nights in Cincinnati to bowl—and we sometimes team up with the guys' league and have seniors' tournaments. One of the widowers I took a liking to, Seymour, who's sixty-eight, seemed to always try to pick me to be on his team (and I'm certainly not *that* good a bowler with my 128 average). Well, we began dating and sleeping over at each other's apartments from time to time—and our sexual encounters were pleasant but not earth-shattering. I read some of those self-help books on how to become more romantic—things like taking a bubble bath together or sipping wine while listening to new-age music, but that kind of stuff just puts us to sleep.

"Anyways, a friend of Seymour's who was on deprenyl gave him a bottle of it, and he began taking it. The result was that it made him as frisky and cocky as a guy half his age. Sleeping together became a whole new experience. I also got some advice from my girlfriend about using these capsules of damiana, ginseng, and avena sativa, which she said were good for making love. After a week, I definitely became more interested in sex too, and it was swell. One night, I suggested that Seymour and I take our pills before going bowling, and they had a much stronger and longer-lasting effect than usual. I think that being active made the effects of our love pills stronger."

"While we bowled that night," Geraldine said, "we were sneakily touching each other under the scoring table, and patting each other's behinds and making each other really excited. We both knew we'd be getting something very special later that night. In the end, it did work out to be really delicious. At our age, it was a fine way to add something new to our sexual repertoire."

Arlene, forty-three, said that she uses exercise and love potions in a different way. She's been a ballet dancer since she was a little girl, and she still constantly keeps up with her stretching and other exercises. "Sometimes I do my bar exercises naked, and my boyfriend really gets off watching me doing those stretches. We take gingko and ginseng every day to prep us up for our lovemaking sessions, so he gets really horny as I bend this way and that. I stretch in ways that tease him, and I don't let him touch me even for a second until I'm completely finished. He just watches and drools. Then I finally give him permission to caress me, and we both go crazy from the built-up sexual tension. I just love it—it's like the song that goes, 'we come in colors everywhere'. We just screw and come and screw and come. What could be finer?"

## Erotic Videos

Aside from exercising, the University of Washington study also showed that one method of increasing a woman's desire for sex is to watch pornography. This was proven when women were attached to lie-detector type equipment that measured their physiological responses to graphic sex films. This heightened sexual readiness can become a perfect backdrop for the use of an aphrodisiac.

Dr. Waldman said, "Couples have told me that watching erotic films while on aphrodisiacs is excellent. Women seem to like these X-rated films as much as men do, although their choice of style is flexible. Some women may prefer a soft-core film like *The Story of O* rather than the hard-core videos. Perhaps a good way to start trying out the mix of aphrodisiacs-plus-eroticism is to rent videos and screen them with your mate."

Roseanne's second husband, Barry, bugged her for a couple of months to watch a porno film with him, but she always demurred. "At first I thought it was kind of revolting to see people's private parts blown up to the size of a TV screen. I'm fifty-four, so I'm not a kid anymore, and I've seen that kind of scene in small glimpses over the years. My first husband used to sneak off with the boys from time to time to play poker while those porno movies played in the background, but it wasn't something that women were interested in. In fact, he'd be smelling of cigarettes and whiskey when he came back home, so it was all a big turnoff.

"My new husband, Barry, who's fifty-one, and I had lovely sex together, and he occasionally cracked open an amyl-nitrate vial and inhaled it to give himself a bigger erection. That was fine with me. I also take a capsule containing dong quai [a Chinese herb] once in a while as it increases my libido."

Roseanne continued, "One night Barry found a comedy-travelogue porno film at the video store and I began watching it with him. It involved a story of a young woman screwing her way through Europe with all types of men and women in all types of situations. I guess I was pleasantly surprised by the fact that I was very interested in it this time around. It must be due to the fact that I like Barry more than my first husband, and that I was already turned on due to the aphrodisiac effects of the dong quai. I wouldn't say the woman porno star was making love—she was fucking anything that walked. She had sex on a tow truck with a mechanic, on a kitchen counter with two chefs, and in a men's locker room with several soccer players simultaneously."

Rosanne added, "Barry took his whiff of his amyl nitrate, and we got naked under the covers as we watched the movie. He caressed my clitoris and vulva for ages while the woman on the screen was sucking cocks and vaginas, kissing other women's breasts, and getting screwed in every direction that could be filmed with a zoom lens. Often the whole screen would fill up with a close-up of genitals and I began imagining it was me doing all the screwing, not her. By the time Barry began fucking me himself, I was ready to explode in orgasm. I squealed almost as loudly as that porno star did when I climaxed! Barry was as pleasantly surprised as I was. I certainly recommend this activity to any woman."

A younger group of couples who had been friends in college were reunited for a forty-fifth birthday party when the host, Paul, showed the old porn movie that several of them had seen on a memorable New Year's Eve twenty-five years earlier. The film, *Behind the Green Door*, came out on the heels of *Deep Throat* and was considered very risqué back then. As an added touch, he and his wife Carly prepared some very special cookies.

Paul said, "It was a kick to see the old movie again and listen to our college friends saying how they learned a lot about sex acts from it. One woman said she even tried anal sex after seeing the movie just to feel what it was like. While the movie was playing on the TV, I handed out cookies Carly and I made with yohimbine, marijuana and damiana leaves that were singed first on a frying pan, and a touch of ambergris. On the TV were naked bodies with full-screen views of giant hard-ons inside giant pussies, and genitals from every angle and in every orifice.

"The fun started when everybody who ate one of our cookies began to act really horny after half an hour. The women were glued to the TV screen, some with their hands in their own laps or their boyfriends', and were saying things like, 'I wonder how much money my husband and I could make by doing one of these?' 'I wonder how it would feel to have so many penises inside me at the same time' and, 'I bet my husband and I would look better than those two. Meanwhile, the guys were saying things like, 'Mine's bigger than his,' and 'Oh honey, you're much better looking than *she* is.

"There was so much sexual tension in the air you could smell it. Couples were so horny you knew they'd be screwing as soon as they could. Two single people who had come alone said they were going to grab a cab together. Many of my friends called to thank me the next day for having such a good time before *and after* the party. It was one of the most successful ways to have a party that I can think of."

Paul added, "Carly and I were both feeling really horny and stoned from those great cookies. So we took off our clothes and propped up a mirror at the head of our bed. Then we watched ourselves just like we were in our own video, screwing and sucking each other in any way possible. We were looking at our reflection while we were screwing doggy style, and she had a great orgasm. We were so turned on we kept right on fucking. For fun, when I came, I pulled out my cock out of her vagina and aimed my hard-on to come all over her ass just like they do in the porno movies. It wasn't very polite, but it sure felt wild.

"All of us had such a good time that we vowed to repeat our performances twenty-five years from now!"

One couple went one step further in the erotica field. They took in a live sex show with "lap dancing" in Toronto—and were very, very pleased. Said Lucie, forty-three, "My husband Kevin and I had stopped in at a health supply store and bought some L-arginine on a lark. We had taken it before, and it had been a very pleasant addition to our sexual passion. We took a couple of capsules after we had some pizza and then kept on walking in the beautiful summer night. We came up to this one place that advertised lap dancing. Both of us were very curious about it, and we thought we'd have a drink and see what it was all about. Luckily, I wasn't the only woman customer there, so I wasn't too conspicuous. The working women inside were knockouts. There were blondes, brunettes, and redheads, all with lovely bodies, and all wandering around the tables. These women were dressed in the most revealing and provocative outfits: baby doll pajamas, see-through negligees, skimpy bras and panties, and even leather thongs. On stage, the women took turns dancing totally naked, spreading their legs wide from time to time like gymnasts."

Lucie continued, "Before long, the working ladies began to approach us. They'd shake our hands, say hello, and sit down and talk for a moment. None asked why I was there, and I was glad they didn't. Although these women were only in it for the money, it was quite intimate to have all these semi-naked women at such close proximity. My husband's eyes were almost bulging out of his head even though he tried to act nonchalant about it all. As for me, I enjoyed looking at all the naked women...

"Another factor in my mind was the possibility of fulfilling a desire I've had for a while. It stems from the fact that I'm very small-breasted, and I've always wanted to touch another woman's large breasts just to see what I was missing. I had discussed it with Kevin, and he just laughed it off. By now, he and I were both tingly from the effects of the L-arginine. We were both pressing against each other and bristling with sexual energy. One lovely, tall, blond woman about twenty-five years old sat down with us and introduced herself as Ursulla. She had really large breasts, a very slim waist, and a nicely rounded bottom, and it was very intriguing to have this lovely creature at our bidding.

"Kevin and I both took to her, and she offered to dance for us together in one of the private booths at the back of the bar. We were quite giddy from the effects of the L-arginine, and that made us braver than we normally are! We simply looked at each other and nodded our eager approval.

"A moment later we gave her some money and followed her to a narrow, very dark room at the back of the place and sat down in a booth the size of a shower stall covered by a flimsy blue velvet curtain. Ursulla took a small blue towel and placed it over Kevin's lap as he and I sat on a large armchair.

"As a new song came over the speakers, Ursulla pulled off her skimpy white bikini bottom and began writhing her naked bum in front of us. She'd turn from time to time, and her neatly trimmed vagina would be right in front of our faces, which made Kevin's eyes grow even larger. But I was more interested in her breasts. Before taking off her top, she turned around and began rubbing her naked butt right on Kevin's lap. She bumped-and-grinded her nicely rounded ass right on top of his towel-covered cock. I gathered that guys are allowed to pull their cocks out of their pants as long as they were covered by the towel, and the woman would keep rubbing against their penises until the guy came. I thought that was a pretty dumb and expensive way for a guy to get his jollies, but who can understand guys anyway?

"Ursulla then got up and took off her top, and her breasts were amazing—large and round, and undulating as she danced to the music. She then straddled both of us, facing forward, and I couldn't contain myself any longer. The effects of the L-arginine and nudity made me absolutely giddy. So I asked Ursulla if I could touch her breasts. She laughed and said she wasn't supposed to, but that I didn't look like a cop. So, as she faced us, I placed my hands on one breast and then the other, manipulating them and then caressing the nipples in my fingertips. Her breasts did feel quite wonderful, softer than I had imagined, and it made me feel very turned on. I think she liked it too, or at least she pretended she did. As I stroked her nipples, they became hard and erect. I liked being able to do that. I could see Kevin had a very big erection under the stupid blue towel, but I wouldn't have allowed him to touch her or vice versa even if either of them wanted to. We enjoyed another close lap dance, and then he and I were so horny that we quickly grabbed a cab home."

Lucie concluded, "We were making out like crazy right in the taxi, and the moment we were home alone, our clothes went flying. We turned around on top of each other to do some sixty-nine, and we were orally pleasing each other and caressing each other everywhere. The whole night turned out to be a beautiful session of foreplay, starting from the moment we took the L-arginine. It was probably the best sexual experience we've ever had. I'm confident we'll top it someday because we're curious and will try something new again. I think Kevin stays satisfied with me because we can enjoy sexual experiences such as this. As for my curiosity about touching a woman's breasts—Ursulla satisfied my desire and made me realize I was happy I didn't have to lug around such large breasts!"

## *Music*

Music also seems to bring out the best in aphrodisiacs. At an anniversary dinner party she held, Rhoda, forty-four, prepared an aphrodisiac punch she invented with the help of a homeopath. The punch contained concentrated tinctures of damiana and muira puama with a touch of ambergris, all mixed into a tangy sangria. Rhoda added dark rum and sprinkled in some powdered gingko biloba for good measure. Said Rhoda, "We started serving the punch before dinner, and people were sipping it all night. It had a deep, earthy, fruity flavor—and it warmed you up as you drank it. I had several nice CD's with danceable music playing in the background.

"By the time we rolled up the carpets, turned up the sound system, and began dancing, everyone had taken on a happy glow. I watched couples as the music played, and they were swaying beautifully to the rhythm in a way I can only describe as dirty dancing! When there was a salsa song, their thighs were deeply embedded in each other's groins, and when there was a slow crooning song by Céline Dion, couples looked like they were glued to each other. There was one gay couple there, and even they were practically making out in front of all of us. Both the men and women were letting their hands roam over their partners' butts, and I decided to turn out the lights for one of the songs. There was lots of groaning and sighing during that song—and two of the couples disappeared upstairs as soon as I turned the lights back on. I admit I peeked into one of the rooms through the keyhole in the bathroom door, but it was only because they were groaning and squealing so much that I became really curious. The two of them were fucking away as if they were part of an Olympic event. It was the most successful party I ever gave."

Getting dressed up is an excellent start for an evening that will feature an aphrodisiac, according to Caitlin, a thirty-six-year-old accountant. She and her husband plan a full night of love, sex, and dancing—and often add an aphrodisiac into the festivities.

Caitlin said, "When my husband Greg and I get invited to a formal event like a charity ball, I really like to make a show of it. Getting dressed up and looking sexy in a big room full of other dressed-up people makes you see yourself and your mate in a different light. I slip into a tight black or red dress with a big slit up the side, and put on some nice red lipstick because it turns my guy on. During the night, Greg and I will pop one or two of the combination capsules containing yohimbine and L-arginine, and we'll get even more turned on. On occasion, we may trade partners on the dance floor with another couple just for one song, and I know that whatever woman's dancing with him is getting off on the feel of his hard-on against her thigh. But we know we always save the best for each other, and we begin touching each other right in the car on the way home.

"When I have a fancy dress on, Greg likes to have sex with me while I'm still wearing it, so he pulls it up to my waist and caresses my vagina inside my panties. Man, it feels so good. I get down on my knees with my dress still on, of course, and I begin sucking on his boner almost as if I'm at an altar and I'm praying. When he finally slides his penis inside me, my vagina feels like it's going to erupt with pleasure. He usually can wait for me to come first, and then he'll move a bit faster and harder so that he comes too, and I feel his hot sperm shooting off into me.

"We'll end up jumping into a hot shower after the first sex session, then pop another capsule—either the same or even a niacin—and by the time we get to bed we're almost ready to start going again. We lie around in bed naked and I rub a bit of ylang-ylang scented cream onto both of our tummies as we caress each other. Greg flips me over when he's ready, and buries his tongue in my cunt again. The second intercourse session is slower, longer, and more serene—but the sensations inside my vagina are also more intense because I'm so primed up. Greg often puts his little finger in my anus at that point while his cock is inside my pussy, and it drives me wild. When I come again it's like taking a trip to the stars. What a rush! I might suck on him and make him come in my mouth because I like it when every orifice is fulfilled. By then, we're so dead tired I don't think any aphrodisiac substance on earth could get us to move anymore, and we pass out all night. What times those are. They make the rest of the week livable!"

## Location, Location, Location

Psychologist Dr. Turkat often advises patients to have sex in strange and different locations to help turn each other on. "It's not very conducive to promoting an active sex life if you get into a routine in which you always have sex, say, every Sunday morning in the same bed. Spontaneity keeps lovemaking exciting and interesting. If using aphrodisiacs turns you on, it's also a good idea to try different ones from time to time. Another idea is to talk dirty when you feel like it. When you act more earthy and sexy it can increase passion and turn on both you and your mate."

One couple took the idea to a bit of an extreme. Charlie wrote, "I tell my wife Janie not to wear underwear some nights when we're going out, and I might pop her whenever I get a hard-on and we're alone—say, in an elevator, or in an empty balcony at the movie theater. We've done it in the car and in the park many, many times, and in countless swimming pools and hot tubs.

"Both of us have developed a habit of drinking damiana tea with bee pollen honey, and it keeps us feeling young and perky. I actually think that this special tea makes Janie's pussy tighter and hotter for my cock. The special tea also keeps me ready to get hard and excited. I like the challenge of Janie's tight pussy because it takes an extra effort to shove my cock into her since I'm really big—but I get so hard from the concept of fucking her spontaneously, and she gets so lubricated from her own horniness, that my boner slips right in. Sometimes I ask Janie if she's decided to become a virgin again because she's so tight, and we laugh. We both usually come quickly—which is just as well because we could get caught if people walked into the semi-private areas we find for screwing. Then, we go about the rest of the evening, like watching the end of the movie or going out for dinner, and we have this feeling of peace and sexiness between us. It's what I call bonding.

"My favorite place to do it with her is in areas where we can see other people but they can't see us. Like if a theater balcony is empty, we sneak up the stairs and go to the back and I get her to bend over the seats, with her bum facing me. Then I can fuck her from behind as we both watch the movie and the people below. We once did it this exact way in a church during Sunday services. We were way in the back of a balcony as the service continued. We both said the right responses, like 'Amen,' when we were supposed to. It was so exciting up there—I don't think Jesus would mind. I mean we are married, after all, and this is a way of making us feel closer and more in love with each other."

Michael and Christina have a rather unusual way to turn

each other on—they go to the zoo and try to see if they can find any animals having intercourse with each other. "It started when our kids were small and we'd take them to the San Diego Zoo near our home," Christine reported. "Michael and I found we just liked watching animals be animals, especially when they're humping each other—it's a real turn-on. Now the kids are teens so they prefer to hang around the mall or whatever, so Michael and I go to the zoo alone. It's so much fun. My sister in Paris sends us these ambergris-coated bonbons which we munch on during our zoo outings. Every once in a while we'll see the bears or lions or otters getting it on with each other or just trying to mount each other. And even if they're not being sexual, when you're at the zoo with all the naked animals it makes you feel animalistic and primitive yourself. The candies add a nice touch because they come from the insides of whales—so we bond with nature and the rest of the animals, in a way. After walking around for a few hours we get back home in the afternoon and lock the bedroom door. Then I turn around backward and get up on my elbows and knees so Michael can hump me from behind. It's great."

Christina added, "One day Michael bought a video of all kinds of animals screwing, and we get turned on from that too. My favorites are the elephants, who have L-shaped penises which move around on their own and which are so heavy they can knock a man out! Imagine getting that beast behind you trying to hump you! Michael also got a bottle of aphrodisiac tincture from China made from all kinds of animal penises and other things. He claims it makes him bigger and harder, and I play along and agree—he certainly acts more horny and animalistic when he's on it, and that's the part I like.

"I reach behind myself between my legs and rub and tickle his testicles while he's humping me, and he starts squealing and grunting. I read somewhere that squeezing the man's balls a bit really empties out all the come from them when he climaxes, and I think that happens to him. Now he always reminds me to tickle his balls if I ever forget, so I know he gets off on that."

Ginette, a French-Canadian woman in her thirties, manufactures scented candles and swears by the aphrodisiac powers of those that are citrus-scented. Her favorite lovemaking location is a bubble bath inside a warm house with a raging snowstorm outside. Ginete said, "I'll light a few dozen lemon-scented candles near the bathtub, add some bubble bath, and invite my man Pierre to come relax with me in the hot, soapy water. I know he loves this scene because he drops whatever he's doing—even if he's watching a hockey game—and takes off all his clothes and comes right in with me. All around us are the flickering scented candles, and we light up a pipeful of yohimbine and pot and lie back against opposite sides of the tub.

"Under the water, our toes nuzzle each other's genitals, and it's really marvellous. I play with his testicles and squeeze his penis between my feet. Meanwhile, he's putting a couple of toes right into my pussy, and my vulvae feel as perky and bright as the soapy bubbles lit up by a thousand flickering pinpoints of candlelight. Once in a while he'll rub the arch of his foot around and around on my soapy breasts and squeeze my nipples in between his toes. Even if there's a terrible winter snowstorm outside, we feel like we're in the Caribbean.

"The total effect of the bubble bath, scented candles, and pipeful of yohimbine is overwhelming. Soon we can't stay even two feet apart any longer, and we slide together. I get up on his lap and aim his penis into my vagina or anus and let him enter me. We just sit there in that position hugging each other for fifteen to thirty minutes. Instead of trying to come there, we wash up, dry off, get into bed, and lick each other until we come in each other's mouths. By then, it certainly doesn't take long!

"I like kissing him with the taste of my pussy on his lips. It shows how much he appreciates me. We'll smoke a little more yohimbine and then do some regular screwing, and we both usually come again. With entertainment and intimacy like that, there's no need to get out into the snowy night for anything!"

A thirty-something couple from Atlanta, Vicky and Jason, use a videocam to play "Fashion TV," explaining that they often spice up their night by sipping a punch made from muira puama, ginseng, and a Jamaican green liqueur called Chartreuse. This liqueur is made from the essences of local roots along with a heavy dash of allspice, and it helps bring out the aphrodisiac qualities of the muira puama. They learned about this punch at their favorite vacation area, Jamaica.

Vicky explained, "My boyfriend Jason and I went on a vacation to Montego Bay, and our little jitney stopped at a local market where this amazing wizened old lady made us lunch of ackee and egg sandwiches washed down by a soursop drink. She winked at me and told me I'd be having a good time that night—and was she ever right, especially in terms of Jason having a good time. I guessed that it was the soursop that gave us the extra sexual urge and the strength to act on it. My guy was really hard and hot and wanted to keep having sex with me half the night. As for me, I've never felt so sexually fulfilled before.

"We made up our minds to see the lady again, and after she hinted that it would be nice to have some American money, she explained that she always puts some strong muira puama tea in the soursop she makes, and that all the couples she sells to come back for more. She sold us some vials of her muira puama tea, and on her instructions, we added it into the Chartreuse that we had at the hotel bar. The effect was twice as strong as with the soursop. It made our Jamaican trip *really* memorable. We had sex three or four times every single day. It was nonstop intercourse. We even did it on the beach on a couple of beautiful starlit nights. Actually, the thing that did slow us down by the end of our trip was the fact that my vagina and Jason's penis were getting worn out from all that screwing."

Vicky added, "Now we make the same mixture ourselves at home in Atlanta with an extra dash of ginseng, and instead of just drinking it and lying around screwing, we play with the video camera as we're sipping away. Jason gets turned on by filming us screwing each other on camera, but I like something more sophisticated like playing Fashion TV.

"Jason films me as I saunter down the pretend-runway with some new blouse or skirt that I bought. Then I come down the runway again, but dressed only in fancy, see-through, sexy underwear. He gets excited filming me, and zooms in on different parts of me—especially my breasts and vagina and butt—but we don't touch each other at all. Then I take the camera and film him doing some runway scenes for me in a pair of his own sexy bikini shorts. Sometimes for a laugh I make him wear my lacy lingerie, including the bra and panties and baby-doll top, and get him to pretend to be me.

As we make our FTV video, he's got a nice, big erection and you can see the outlines of it bursting out against his shorts or whatever he's wearing. So I zoom in on that part of him. Finally, we play the scenes of ourselves on our big-screen TV, and we are more than ready to start fucking. The visual foreplay works fantastically, and the heartwarming drink we learned about from our Jamaican friend primes both of us perfectly for scream-level orgasms."

One couple reported that their location is so bad that they're forced to masturbate! The two of them are separated for months at a time, but they've found a new way to make out with each other using "virtual sex." Larry explained, "I bought two of those little cameras that you plug into your computer for Bunky and myself, so that we can actually see each other when we do live e-mail together. She's working as a nurse on a reservation for a year, and we can only meet every couple of months, so we masturbate as we watch each other on our computer monitors. It's a way of staying intimate with each other. We start off by talking to each other as we watch each other on the monitor. Since we need a bit of stimulation to get us started, we take some niacin and that makes us start to tingle. I tease Bunky by getting her to show me her breasts and then her pussy on the screen. I like to watch as she tugs at her nipples and clitoris with her fingers, and then rubs her pussy hard with the palm of her hand. Meanwhile, I aim my own camera at my hard-on as I play with myself, and I make sure she can see the jism shooting out into a tissue when I come. The computerized virtual sex keeps us hot for each other. When we do meet for the first time after separating, we'll take some niacin to make us feel like we do when we're talking to each other on our computers, and we have real-life fireworks."

### Miscellaneous Tricks

Just plain talking dirty is a real turn-on for a couple from South Dakota. Noreen said, "Gerry hardly talks to me at all, but if we smoke a mixture of pot and damiana, he just starts talking nonstop—and it quickly becomes really dirty. He starts by whispering sweet stuff into my ear about how I'm his 'little dogie' and after a little while it becomes, 'Wouldn't you like to have my cock inside your sweet pussy right now?' or 'Come close little darling, I want to feel the heat from your cunt on me.' I guess I love him because I even love hearing the dumb sexy things he says. It turns me on.

"I start to think, 'Yeah, my pussy really is hot,' and, 'Yeah, I really would like his boner inside my vagina,' and 'I really do want to feel him coming inside my mouth.' It doesn't sound so great though, unless I've gotten all stimulated from the damiana and pot. I've told my girlfriends to try those special joints with their husbands, and a couple of them said that they got some really good sex too after smoking this combination. Plus you sleep really well after it."

A truly unusual turn-on that we don't recommend comes from Roberta, twenty-nine, and her boyfriend Ned, thirty-nine. Ned reported, "We were out for a walk at San Francisco's Fisherman's Wharf in the afternoon when we stumbled onto the Medieval Dungeon, a torture museum. We had just smoked a joint and taken some capsules of avena sativa, and were feeling really good. We had passed it a million times before without ever considering going in there. It was only something for tourists, after all. Anyway, it was a rainy day, so we thought we'd look at the crazy stuff inside there. There were about one hundred truly horrible sights.

"There were life-size mannequins of men and women being tortured in terrible, humiliating ways with horrible instruments. Also, there were very detailed drawings showing ways to kill people while causing them tremendous pain and degradation. Like sawing them in two, or slowly squishing their heads open in a vice, or breaking them on the wheel. You really wonder how mankind can ever be so sick and cruel as to produce this type of depravity.

"Roberta and I felt sick and disgusted by it all. We went back to my place, and we were both really upset. We felt nauseated and nervous from those sights, and we just clung together for emotional support as our hearts beat fast from the stress of it all. But something happened. While we were nervous and jittery, we were also feeling very horny. I think we wanted the comfort of sex to get us over the emotional agony of our experience. Sort of like something bad had happened to us, and we needed each other for support."

Ned continued, "We started caressing each other's genitals and then screwing each other. It was so very hot and comforting. We clutched each other tightly to make sure our genitals were as close together as could be. So feeling bad turned around into feeling really, really good. We waited a long time with my cock inside her before having orgasms because the clinging together was so satisfying.

"I guess seeing a horror movie could have had the same effect. It's funny but true. I was glad we had taken the pot and the avena sativa, because our orgasms were truly extraordinary that day. And we felt much closer as a couple because of the way we were able to help each other soothe our nerves and release our anxieties through sex."

## Spiritual Aspects of Aphrodisiac Use

"A common theme emerges from the couples who develop ways of turning their partners on," Dr. Turkat pointed out. "They're really finding ways of turning themselves on at the same time. A perfect example of this can be seen in the couple who shared the bubble bath with scented candles. The woman was turning herself on with this foreplay, and her excitement turned on her partner. This is also true for the couple that used the video camera to take videos of each other as each pretended to be a fashion model. They enjoyed seeing good-looking videos of themselves walking down their fashion runway, and this was part of the ritual that turned them on.

"Looking in from the outside, you may say that it's narcissistic, but it's the sharing aspect that's truly important. When they share their fantasies and aren't afraid to expose their inner selves to each other, a deeper bond develops. It's a spiritual connection involving trust, openness, sharing, and their own human frailties. These couples have found ways to be spiritually connected partly through the use of their sexual connection."

In fact, since the dawn of recorded history, people have been fascinated with finding new ways to incite and sustain their sexual drive. The ancient Babylonians experimented with various plant preparations six thousand years ago to increase their sex drives. People have been consulting medicine men, priests, and shamans about sexual stimulants ever since they came into being. Modern-day psychological studies have shown that the average man or woman thinks about specific sex acts about a hundred times a day. It's one more proof that our sexuality is deeply ingrained in our spirit. There's no reason to doubt that our caveman ancestors and all those who've populated the planet since then have been as preoccupied with sex as we are. Sexuality is part of who we are, part of our spirituality.

How is this yearning for sexual gratification helped by the use of aphrodisiacs? Let's turn to some startling statistics. A federally funded study called the Massachusetts Male Aging Study of men between forty and seventy concluded that 52 percent of them reported some degree of impotence—and that adds up to more than fifty million American men. Among the forty-year-olds, 5 percent noted they had complete impotence as did 15 percent of the seventy-year-olds, for a total of twenty million men.

As for women, research indicates that at least this same amount are dissatisfied with the way their own bodies respond to sex. Dr. Waldman from Montreal commented, "The fact that women can have sex without having to produce an erection disguises the fact that many of them aren't satisfied with their sex lives. Woman are far more reluctant to complain to doctors about sexual unhappiness than men are. Women have a right to enjoy their sex lives just as much as men do, and exploring their sexuality with aphrodisiacs may be a way to promote their own satisfaction."

The spiritual need to have satisfactory sex can be aided through the use of substances that encourage sexual relations to thrive. As noted previously, using aphrodisiacs can spice up your sex life and make your relationship with your mate closer and more vibrant. Feeling good sexually has added benefits—people live an average of ten years longer if they're having regular sex!

# 3

# Herbal and Plant Aphrodisiacs

In this chapter, we've concentrated on the traditional herbal and plant preparations that seem to be the most popular and effective. There are dozens of other substances that are also being sold in America, and we hope this guide will serve as a basis for comparison and exploration. There's quite a lot to try right here though! These items can be obtained in their natural form or in more concentrated liquid extracts, tinctures, and potions.

### Yohimbine

Yohimbine is the active ingredient derived from the corklike interior bark of the corynanthe yohimbe tree. It has been used to boost sexual prowess in both men and women for centuries. The large yohimbe tree, which grows in the steamy forests of West Africa, has been coveted by natives of Africa and the West Indies as the source of an important drug used in rituals and mating ceremonies. Some of the native ceremonies involved intense sexual activity which continued for days or weeks, with much trading of partners, spurred on by the effects of yohimbine. Natives prepared an aphrodisiac concoction by making a concentrated tea from this interior bark. They simmer an ounce of it in a quart of water for twenty minutes, then strain and drink.

In recent years in the United States, yohimbine has been refined into a prescription drug that has been approved by the FDA for treatment of impotence. In fact, it's the only herb that the FDA has approved for such treatment. While you can obtain a doctor's prescription for it, you can also readily buy it in its natural form or as a tincture called yohimbine hydrochloride in most health food stores and in ordinary drugstores.

Physiologically, yohimbine is known to produce excellent enhancement of sexual desire, prowess, and enjoyment. It acts by stimulating the spinal nerves at the level of receptor sites and by boosting neurotransmitter levels. It also increases blood flow into the genitalia, thus making it a sex enhancer for both men and women, and may produce elevated blood pressure and heart rate.

Physiologically, for a penis to stay hard the blood rushing into it through the connected arteries has to be trapped in the erectile tissues by a simultaneous tightening of the veins— and that's what yohimbine does. In fact, veterinarians have even administered yohimbine to stallions who are reluctant to mate as a means of making them more inclined to breed.

While yohimbine is not powerful enough to create an

## Herbal and Plant Aphrodisiacs

erection in men with serious medical problems, it improves sexual function in more than half of men who are able to have some form of sexual activity. Importantly, yohimbine also has a positive sex-enhancing effect on most people taking antidepressants, who commonly experience a drop in libido.

Yohimbine, however, should not be taken in large quantities. Too much can over stimulate the body and cause palpitations or nausea.

What does all this mean to the average couple? One fellow reported that his erections become "as hard as steel" and that yohimbine increased the force and volume of his ejaculation tremendously.

April and Stewart, a couple in their thirties, went on a one-week learn-to-ski vacation in Park City, Utah, and experimented with yohimbine there. Stewart wrote, "We're a normal couple from the Midwest, married for five years, and we get along well most of the time. One reason we picked a ski vacation was to do something different to spice up our relationship. We started out learning to do the snowplow in all that deep snow, and it made us dead tired the first couple of days. We both fell asleep without even a kiss goodnight. By the third day we were a bit more energetic, and we were able to walk around the main street in town. We found that it was pretty health oriented. There were posters and flyers everywhere offering such things as Rolfing massage, colon irrigation, and 'fantastic herbal remedies.' For a lark we visited a health food store hoping to find something to alleviate our sore muscles, and the clerk ended up selling us a bottle of yohimbine tincture, saying it would increase both mine and April's vitality. I found out later that 'vitality' was a codeword for libido. This was all new to us but we figured it couldn't hurt since the guy we bought it from must have been a Mormon, so we each took several drops daily mixed in with our orange juice.

"The effects came two days later. Much to our delight, when April and I went to the hotel whirlpool to stretch out our sore muscles after a tough day of skiing, my cock became erect and hard as a ski pole. Those spontaneous erections were to continue for the entire rest of our vacation, even while skiing with the cold wind blowing through my legs. There were other guests in the whirlpool, but they couldn't see my hard-on (luckily) because of the turbulence. For fun I took April's hand underwater and placed it on top of my bathing suit, and she practically burst out laughing. I eventually snuck out of the whirlpool, staying close behind April so no one would notice my condition. Back in our room, April practically jumped me. She said, 'I was so relieved that you were excited because I've been practically climbing the walls out of frustration for the past two days. I didn't want to pressure you to have sex when you seemed so tired, but *this* is a different story!'"

Stewart added, "The yohimbine made us horny for the entire rest of the trip, and for the rest of the time it took us to finish the bottle. It didn't matter how exhausted we got from skiing, we'd screw like rabbits whenever we got back alone—even while standing up in the shower.

"For me, I felt like my ejaculations were more powerful than ever, while April said that it was much easier for her to come than ever before. She said her whole body felt tingly, from her spine to her vulva. When I did enter her, she was always really lubricated, and she seemed to be shivering from excitement. Even her breasts felt more luscious and sexy. Every time I caressed them she shuddered. We knew that the

O.J. spiked with the yohimbine tincture was making us both become more sensitive and responsive.

"One morning, we did oral sex on each other before we got out of our nice warm bed, and we came in each other's mouths in such powerful, heart-stopping gushes that we laughed about our passion the whole day. On our last day, we skipped our ski lesson and just hung around inside our hotel room naked, having a truly memorable day of screwing and caressing. I was glad we found out how delightful something like yohimbine could be as an addition to our normal lovemaking routine. It kind of made it feel like a little celebration."

A couple who moved to Taunton, Massachusetts, from Boston were despondent about their boring weekends until they tried a yohimbine mixture. Carson said, "There's not much to do in Taunton on the weekend except to play Bingo or visit the silversmith factory, so for kicks my wife, Vanna, and I try anything different. The video stores do stock a lot of porno movies, so we'd get a few of them and watch them at double speed after we put the kids to bed. It's fun seeing all that quick-moving, energetic, full-screen screwing. The video clerk noticed us getting these flicks a few times, and he suggested we pick up these herbal capsules that had a mix of yohimbine and avena sativa, saying they'd increase our appreciation for the flicks. Vanna and I began taking the caps on Friday. By the time we were ready to watch the movies Saturday night, we had developed a very special, sensitive feeling all over our skin. We also opened a couple of caps and spread them into a joint before we rolled it and smoked it. That made us even more mellow.

"On the TV screen was the regular gang of anonymous naked women and men rubbing suntan lotion on each other and then sucking and screwing each other. But they suddenly seemed very attractive to both of us. There were penises, tongues, and fingers sliding in and out of orifices and glistening with body fluids. My own penis became so hard and thick I couldn't stand it. Vanna was all hot beside me. I could feel her rubbing her breasts on my back, and I was suddenly dying to get her naked."

Carson continued, "In a moment I began licking and sucking on her cunt, and I wanted to swallow every drop of her juices. She tasted so wild and sexy, and she was groaning and screeching with every stroke of my tongue. I turned around and she began sixty-nining me, but her mouth just didn't seem big enough.

"I wanted my cock deep inside something, so I began poking it into her juicy wet vagina. It was some of the wildest and horniest sex we've ever had. When I came, it felt like I was a geyser shooting out sperm. We lay there for a while watching the porno stars as they kept on screwing, and before we knew it, I got hard again, so I flipped Vanna over and began screwing her doggy-style. I reached around and played with her clit in my fingers, and we both came simultaneously, grunting and groaning. It was really hot and wild, man, and it was quite a way to spend a night."

One woman from Mystic, Connecticut, swears that using yohimbine along with a combination of scents is the best natural aphrodisiac available. "I bought some musk-scented massage oil and some Indian incense from a small store, and I began laying my trap. My goal was to snare this dentist I met at work," confessed Kendra, thirty-seven. "He was cute even though he was around fifty, and his name was Eduardo.

"We had gone out together for pizza a couple of times, but he acted very aloof toward me. So I invited him over for

## Herbal and Plant Aphrodisiacs

dinner and told him to bring a bottle of wine. I lit the incense in my apartment an hour before he arrived, and it had a really exotic smell. Then I rubbed some of the musk oil on myself, and the smell of that on my warm skin was getting me really turned on. When Eduardo came in, I got him to sit down on the sofa and I rubbed some of the massage oil on his shoulders and neck. That got him to begin warming up to me right away in an emotional sense."

Kendra continued, "I steeped yohimbine in boiling water to make a tea out of it, added two capsules of Siberian ginseng, and blended it all together with honey. It looked pretty muddy, and it also tasted sort of muddy, but I told Eduardo that if we both drank it, it would be good for our health since it came from a health food store. We both gulped down a few mouthfuls and chased it with some plain red wine. I felt a warmth starting from inside my belly, like I had a lightbulb glowing inside me.

"I began to notice a strong bulge in Eduardo's pants. I knew *something* was definitely happening. I'm sure the combination of the musk and incense must have made the special drink work even better. I mean, just one sniff of all that stuff would make anyone feel lusty. We snuggled a bit together, and we didn't even get to start eating the pasta before we began making out like crazy on the floor. I pretended to be a little coy, and he seemed so desperately hard and horny that I let him take off my clothes and then his. I certainly didn't want him to come in his jeans! I grabbed a condom from my drawer, and we began making love in the hottest, sweetest way. I made sure he didn't come fast by holding onto his butt and making him go in a very slow rhythm. I knew I was going wild, and it looked like he was too.

"When he climaxed it was very moving and he hung on to

me really, really tight, squeezing my ass in his strong dentist's hands. He caressed my clitoris with his long fingers, and I came a few seconds later. We kissed a bit before putting on our shirts and having the pasta I made. It was a mild night, and we went for a walk over the bridge after dinner. He put his arm around my shoulder in the nicest way and told me he felt very close to me and that he really enjoyed my company. He said he liked the fact that I wasn't trying to pressure him, although maybe secretly I was!"

Kendra added, "The thought did cross my mind as to whether he was especially horny for me or whether he would have wanted to screw any woman who was there after swallowing those aphrodisiacs. I figured I'd find out by seeing if he called me or not. I also figured that if I was enjoying this experience so much with him, he must be enjoying it too with me. He did call me the next day saying he was thinking of me—and we've been seeing each other for six months already. I often change aphrodisiacs, and I also change the scents I use on myself and in my apartment. I think all of this helps maintain the intrigue and mystery between us. And I think our romance will continue, since it started so memorably."

## *Damiana*

Damiana is a shrub that grows wild in Mexico, Bolivia, the West Indies, and South America. In the United States, it's found in Texas, and it's also being cultivated in California. The leaves of this plant act as a powerful aphrodisiac, especially for women, although men are very happy using it as well. Even its botanical name, *Turnera diffusa aphrodisiaca,* takes account of its aphrodisiac properties.

Damiana's erogenous effects stem from the fact that it's a powerful nerve stimulant for the sex organs due to the presence of several alkaloids—and it boosts the circulation. For centuries in Mexico, women have been using it in drinks for themselves as a prelude to lovemaking. They'll prepare a tea from damiana by boiling two heaping tablespoons of the leaves in water for five minutes, or they'll soak a handful of leaves in tequila or vodka for a week for its active ingredients to infuse the alcohol. Since the leaves are rather bitter, honey is often added as a sweetener. In herbal outlets in the United States, damiana is most often found in powdered form in capsules, or already prepared as a liquid tincture or extract. (Note that an extract is five to ten times more powerful than a tincture.) You can simply make your own preferred drink from whichever damiana preparation you obtain and sip it a couple of hours before your expected acts of passion. Start with the extract to find out which form works best for you—and use a recommended brand.

As an added bonus, some partakers of this love potion experience a euphoria while under its influence, similar to getting mildly high on marijuana. Damiana has also been reported to elicit erotic thoughts and dreams in women, adding to its amorous effects. Some reports say that damiana acts as a tonic for the prostate muscle and is a nutrient for the adrenals and sex organs. Along with yohimbine and muira puama, damiana is one of the most popular herbal aphrodisiacs in the world.

Larry, forty-nine, reported that his girlfriend's vagina *tasted* better after the two of them began taking damiana. Larry said, "Aside from the excellent aphrodisiac effects damiana tea had on my girlfriend Theresa and me, I soon noticed that her snatch was tasting really nice when I went down on her—it sort of had the flavor of newly cut grass. She always had a pretty good kind of flavor, something like a mixture of lemon and basil. But the damiana got rid of the tart-lemony part, so it was nicer.

"The combination of the new flavor and the extra sensations we were getting in our sex organs made our oral sexual episodes dynamite. Her lips going up and down my cock felt like they were full of static electricity, like they were making little sparks. And then each time she flicked the tip of her tongue on the little slit at the end of my cock I went wild—it felt like a whiplash of ecstasy on my super-sensitive organ.

"By the time I climax inside her mouth I'm so turned on that my whole body undulates with each spurt of come. Since I'm usually doing cunnilingus on her at the same time, the excitement makes me stick my tongue right into her pussy as far as I can, and that usually is the coup de grace to make her climax too. She has this nice-tasting gush of come herself, with that grassy flavor, and that turns me on even more. I only have to wait about twenty minutes before I get hard again and begin fucking her the regular way. It was great to learn about this type of aphrodisiac. It's one of the best things we've tried."

## *Avena Sativa*

Avena sativa is an extract of wild green oats that is known to have aphrodisiac properties for both men and women. A study by the Institute for Advanced Study of Human Sexuality in California showed that 50 percent of women taking avena sativa had an increase in the number of orgasms they experienced and in the amount of vaginal lubrication produced in response to sexual stimuli. Another study at Budapest University indicated that men experienced greater sexual stamina and drive when taking avena sativa. Other researchers found that this substance has the effect of raising testosterone levels in both women and men up to 187 percent.

While avena sativa has a libido-enhancing effect, especially on people who have low testosterone levels, it seems to have its most important benefits as a booster to increase the effects of other aphrodisiacs. It's often found in formulations of aphrodisiacs containing stronger substances like yohimbine, damiana, or L-arginine. For instance, one common preparation contains capsules with 135 milligrams avena sativa, 157 milligrams damiana, and 157 milligrams of the herb urtica dioica.

You may find it beneficial to buy an extract of avena sativa to drizzle into other aphrodisiacs you may be trying. Jim, fifty-eight, noted, "I enjoy ordering my own custom mixtures from the herbal store. Some of the items I buy regularly are dong quai, muira puama, Siberian ginseng, sarsaparilla, bee pollen, zinc, damiana, and avena sativa. I'll mix some of these products together in various combinations to see what effects are produced. I think that changing the proportions often means that my girlfriend and I won't get accustomed to any substance and thus require more of it to create an effect."

A thirty-seven-year-old woman from Oakland, Angie, planned a weekend trip to the Sonoma Valley's vineyards with her boyfriend and brought along capsules containing a strong blend of avena sativa. "A girlfriend of mine recommended taking avena sativa because she was able to be multiorgasmic when she was on it, and she said guys are supposed to get off better on it too. My boyfriend, Marven, was happy to give it a try, so I took it with us as we drove up. We toured three beautiful wineries and took one of the avena sativa caps along with the samples of wine they gave us to try. It made us feel great, really relaxed and definitely very romantic. Before checking in at our motel, we stopped in at one of those mud bath places, and that's where a lot of things happened. We both became really horny as we lay in the piles of steaming hot volcanic ash they use. I think the heat had a multiplier effect on the aphrodisiac we were taking because we both felt very intense. After an attendant hosed us down, we went into the hot spring pool they had adjacent to the mud baths. Luckily, we were going to be alone for half an hour to relax, according to the attendant. Marven floated over to me, and he had one of the hugest erections I have ever seen.

"He began caressing my breasts under the hot water, squeezing them and rubbing them. My breasts felt so wonderful as he touched me, and I almost had an orgasm just from that. The sexual sensations that were building up inside me were incredible. My breasts and vagina were yearning to be touched and manipulated forever."

Angie continued, "I was holding onto the ladder from behind me to keep from sinking in the deep pool, and I spread my legs wide for Marven underwater. I was desperate for him to stick his cock deep into me. He definitely had the exact same idea as I did, and he came right at me with his hips thrust forward and stuck his penis right into my waiting vagina. I was really lubricated so Marven was able to get his cock into me with hardly any trouble even though we were underwater. He wasn't talking, but the expression on his face looked really happy, almost as if he was lost in space, like a doggy who's just mounted another dog and is screwing away.

I thought it was kind of endearing. Both of us hung onto the ladder tightly so we wouldn't float apart while we were screwing. We rubbed our chests together really hard as we screwed, and my ass was banging against the ladder but it didn't matter.

"The sensations of his erection inside my vagina were incredible, and I climaxed in wonderful pulses. I still felt really horny—instead of feeling overly sensitive as I normally do after coming—so I knew I was going to come again. I told Marven to move real slow so he wouldn't come too soon. He did that for a while, but then he couldn't hold back anymore and he began fucking me fast and hard. I knew that was going to be it for him, so I tensed my vaginal muscles and tilted my hips to try to make myself come too. It didn't work again for me, but he was practically screaming when he shot off his cannon. It was all we could do to get our hearts to calm down and try to look normal so we could pretend nothing had happened when the attendant came back.

"For the final segment of our treatment, the attendant wrapped Marven and me in these hot sheets and towels so we almost couldn't move. Once again, we were going to be left alone for fifteen minutes on some cots. Marven, being very debonair, stuck his hand down inside my towel wrappings and played with my vulva and clitoris until I came. This time I was really drenched with vaginal fluids, and it felt great. Marven told me with a laugh that his hand was going to smell of pussy for the whole weekend! We didn't have sex that night because we just passed out. The next day we also took the avena sativa during our tour, and we made excellent love in our motel. We both had a couple of orgasms that day as well during our love sessions. It was quite a vacation weekend to remember."

## Muira Puama

Muira puama, an aphrodisiac made from the roots and bark of a tree growing in the Amazon, is the basis of the Voodoo Ecstasy Cocktail sold in German sex shops. A few drops of the liquid extract mixed with alcohol produces a cocktail that stimulates the sex organs and helps beat the sexual blues. Like many of the other herbal aphrodisiacs, it has a long pedigree, having been used for sexual enhancement for centuries by Brazilian natives, among others.

One of the better ways of preparing it in its raw form is to heat half a quart of sake or vodka almost to the boiling point along with a handful of the powdered bark and roots mixture. Then strain and drink. Muira puama is considered to be weaker than yohimbine, but more of it can be taken without feeling side effects. (Yohimbine, in excessive quantities, can lead to nausea and palpitations.) It's often found in preparations of capsules combining several of these aphrodisiacs, and in Brazil is often mixed with a herbal tonic called catuaba.

While on a business trip, Conrad, fifty-six, went into one of the omnipresent German sex boutiques and bought a vial of Black Magic potion—similar to the Voodoo brand—that contained muira puama. On top of that, the saleswoman sold him niacin capsules and told him to take one along with a dropperful of the Black Magic prior to sex. "I invited my assistant Veronica up to my hotel room for a drink before dinner, and I mixed a couple of screwdrivers," Conrad confessed. "I didn't tell her that I also stirred into them the Black Magic potion plus the crushed-up niacin pills. I was hoping something hot would happen. I was actually dying to have her. She had such beautiful long legs, curly black hair, deep blue eyes, and a great figure. I was secretly praying that the aphrodisiac mixture would do something to turn her on—and I hit the jackpot. It actually turned me on more too."

Conrad noted, "When we finally began walking back to the hotel, after a dinner with our clients, she put her arm in mine and kept saying what a beautiful night it was. This time, she invited me to her room for a nightcap. I stood around close to her as she mixed some gin and tonics, and then—waoh, it all started. She hung onto my arm and stepped right up to me and pressed her breasts right against my chest. That was enough for me to get started too."

An American couple who went to work in Embrapa, Brazil, got caught up in the fervor of muira puama-laced cocktails. The couple, Ellen and Bob, happily reported that the year they spent there was remarkable in terms of the amount of sex they had. Ellen said, "Bob and I had been married for almost ten years, and sex had become a routine once-a-week kind of thing. I would have preferred more than that but he wasn't interested—and, in any case, he found that it made him tired. But after being in Embrapa for a few weeks, things rapidly changed for the better. We started being invited to those all-night dance parties and drinking those punches they always served. I thought it was just the alcohol that made everyone so wild, but I later found out it was the muira puama they were adding to it. Bob and I would be dancing and we'd be hornier than hell the whole night. Bob had a hard-on most of the time as we danced and drank. We couldn't act too wild in public because we were linked to an American university research project, but as soon as we'd get back to our cottage the action would begin.

"We'd throw off our clothes—which would be dripping

with sweat from the dancing and the heat—and start animalistically pressing our bodies and faces against each other. We'd both be so drenched from the dancing and jumping around that we'd actually be sliding around against each other as we writhed together.

"My pussy would be so hot and slippery from my natural juices that his cock could slide right into me from any direction he pleased. I think that was how I discovered I had a G-spot about an inch inside my vagina at the top. I was lying on my back on the floor with Bob kneeling down between my legs and screwing me very energetically. He had to hold onto my waist and hips to keep me from sliding away. He tilted my hips upward at just the right angle, and that put the end of his uncircumcised cock right against this newly found pleasure center, my G-spot. I gasped out in surprise at that moment, and he thought he had hurt me and was going to stop screwing—but I made sure he just kept on thumping his cock into me from the same angle, right against my G-spot. I soon felt like I was having my own simultaneous double climax, one from my clitoris and one from my G-spot, and it was truly mind-boggling."

Ellen added, "During the rest of our stay in northern Brazil, we had many more gut-wrenching sex sessions, almost on a daily basis. Bob got a lot of erections during the day, and he was always really keen to use them in me. The frequency of sex was really amazing. I don't think he was having better orgasms—just more of them, which definitely pleased him. And he never did complain of being tired anymore after screwing. I only realize now that we're back in the States how different we were down there, and that I had better figure out how to make up our own punch of muira puama. Also, I believe the Brazilian women used to add some of this aphrodisiac into a potato-based dish they served called vatapa, and I plan to make that as well. That was such great sex—even better than when we were newlyweds."

## Gingko Biloba

Gingko biloba, usually just referred to as gingko, is one of the products most prescribed by physicians in Europe and Asia, and it's now becoming very popular in North America as well. It's an extract made from the leaves of one of the oldest species of trees on the planet—trees that were around at the same time as the dinosaurs. The tree is native to China and Japan, and now also flourishes in the United States.

As reported in a study by the New York Institute for Medical Research among others, gingko has beneficial psychological effects on most people, including stroke patients, patients suffering from Alzheimer's, and people with problems involving cognitive functions and social behavior. Gingko increases blood and oxygen flow through the brain, and its active ingredient, Egb, acts to regulate the flow of free radicals in the brain and thus to control brain cell damage caused by Alzheimer's. Now millions of people have begun taking gingko to become mentally sharper and to stave off senility.

Many people have also reported that the drug boosts their desire for sex and their ability to have better sex. In fact, it has been found that along with gingko's ability to improve brain circulation, it also increases blood flow to the penis. In a study investigating gingko's effectiveness as an aphrodisiac, 78 percent of men who were unable to have erections due to poor penile blood flow regained their prowess after a few weeks on gingko.

"My brother and I, both widowed, began taking gingko regularly because we believed it would help prevent senility," said Dotty, seventy-six. "We found that it calmed our nerves and that we were able to play thinking games like Scrabble with greater depth and ease. After a couple of months, my brother, Max announced that he was planning to ask one of my friends on a date. I was shocked. It was the first time he even brought up such a concept since his wife died two years ago. He said he felt so good that he didn't want to waste his energy by staying indoors too much."

Dotty added, "My girlfriend, Rae, did start dating him, and a few weeks later she reported that she was delighted that a man of Max's age was willing and able to satisfy her in every way. I'm sure it was the gingko that initiated this amorous behaviour. If any man plans to start asking me out, I'll certainly advise him to start on gingko as well."

Lionel, a retired shipfitter, reported that he and his girlfriend stumbled upon a gingko-and-ginseng combination capsule when they went on a cruise to Hong Kong. "The crowded market stalls were chock-a-block with the strange animals that people eat there and with herbal stores. Ginette and I finally stopped in a friendly-looking place where the owner gave me a knowing nod and sold me this gingko-ginseng mixture to take. Before the end of our Oriental cruise, I began to feel and think better, and then my cock just started to work better too, all by itself. I was getting more and more hard-ons. Ginette's twenty years younger than me at forty-six, and she almost started to complain that I wanted too much sex.

"As our cruise continued I kept on taking the stuff, and I was constantly horny for her. I really appreciate her queen-size body because I'm so skinny and bony. So getting lots of hard-ons was great because I could fuck her even more than normal. It's great to sink into her arms, and to play with her large, round breasts and her big, beautiful ass, and then to actually fuck her and come inside her tight vagina. I love to have her under my control as I pump her between her legs."

Lionel noted, "A couple of times when she wasn't into penetration, she put a lot of hand cream in between her breasts and held them close together while I rubbed my hard-on between them until I ejaculated. Man, that was a pleasure. She has magnificent breasts, and when she holds them like that for me to pleasure myself it's a real turn-on. I started giving her those gingko and ginseng caps, but I don't know yet whether it'll work for her too. These days, she's the one who has to worry about whether or not she can keep up with me, instead of the other way around."

## Dong Quai

Millions of Chinese attest to the aphrodisiac qualities of this herbal product made from the root of a plant that grows widely in China. For women, its aphrodisiac effects arise from the fact that it dilates blood vessels and sensitizes the uterine muscles. In men, it dilates the blood vessels and sensitizes the smooth muscle tissue inside the penis. Aside from enhancing sexual activity, it's widely prescribed to treat painful menstruation and the symptoms of menopause.

Dong quai is usually sold as a liquid extract, with a few drops being taken in water before meals. It's often found in mixtures of women's aphrodisiacs.

Melanie, a sixty-two-year-old woman who recommends dong quai, first started using it when she wanted an alternative to estrogen therapy—and then she noticed the aphrodisiac effects. "I was prescribed the estrogen patch by my doctor to alleviate the effects of menopause, and in fact it did make me feel better by regulating my moods and by making sex more enjoyable. Prior to taking it, I'd use a lubricant before having sex with my husband. But I was reading a bit about how estrogen can increase the risk for breast cancer, which is what my mother died of. When a homeopath recommended that I use dong quai instead of estrogen, I figured why not?."

Melanie added, "Taking dong quai did keep me feeling good, and then, after a couple of weeks, I began to notice that sex felt much better. My vagina and clitoris felt more sensitive and receptive to my husband, and I had orgasms more often. When I thanked my homeopath for his advice, he suggested that my husband try it too. We were surprised because we thought that if it would work for a woman, it would have an antiaphrodisiac effect on a man. But no—my husband's erections became longer lasting, and stiffer. He's also very pleased with the effects. I'm sure we'll be able to keep on having satisfactory sex for another ten years or even more.

"One big change this has had in our sex lives is that since we're now confident about our sexual enjoyment and prowess, we can be more casual about having sex. We went to visit my daughter and our grandchildren up at the cottage in Maine during the summer, and we had sex practically every morning. I know the old bed was creaking and the walls were thin, but we had such a good time having intercourse we didn't care about the noise. I told my daughter we were doing our back exercises in bed before getting up—and she believed me. Children have so much to learn!"

A younger woman with painful menstrual cramps also tried taking dong quai. Nora, twenty-eight, said,"I saw all these weird Chinese herbalist stores on a trip to San Francisco, so I decided to stop in at one on Stockton St. The herbalist recommended a combination of herbs, the prime one being dong quai, that I was supposed to steep as a tea and then drink. The result was that the dong quai seemed to relax my uterus so I didn't get that painful gripping feeling inside me all the time. It also made me feel sexy again during my periods. For the first time I was able to have sex and enjoy it with my boyfriend during that time of the month. We do it when I'm not bleeding heavily, and I even have a nice orgasm sometimes. It was a lot different from lying around scrunched up and telling him not to touch me at all during those days."

# 4

# The New Pharmacological Substances

## The "Magic" Erection Pills

### SILDENAFIL, PHENTOLAMINE, AND APOMORPHINE

In just the past decade, treatment of erectile dysfunction has progressed more than it has in centuries. Most of the traditional herbal and animal aphrodisiacs we've been discussing have been used for thousands of years. Sales of these substances are measured in the hundreds of millions of dollars a year worldwide. Since aphrodisiacs are such big business, anyone who can come up with a new product that's really effective can also cash in. Hence, major drug companies have turned their attention to developing new patented substances that will set them apart from the rest.

For instance, as soon as one of the major American drug companies began releasing details of successful tests for a new erection pill, its stock price almost doubled within the year. By 1997, another company's stock rose sevenfold from its 1993 initial public offering.

This is not to say that the pills are the best choice for every man. Experts point out that many men with serious erectile dysfunction would find better results with injection therapy, intraurethra pellets, an implant, or even a rub-on cream—all of which are already available.

To obtain the pills prior to their being fully approved by the FDA, doctors may be able to obtain them as part of a study or by claiming that a patient needs them to treat another medical condition such as high blood pressure. This practice of prescribing a drug to treat an ailment it wasn't designed for in the first place is called "off-label" use. Many Americans are clamoring to get these pills now through their doctors, thus showing how many people believe they can benefit from an erection brought about by a "magic pill."

Dr. James Barada, a director of the Center for Male Sexual Health in Albany, New York, explained, "There are twenty million American men with erectile dysfunction, and that means there are forty million Americans who want to find a solution, if you include their partners." Dr. Barada pointed out that there has been a major shift in emphasis in pinpointing the origins of this problem. "Whereas in the fifties and sixties most medical experts thought problems were mainly in your head, we now know that only 10 percent of cases are psychological, 30 percent stem from vascular problems of the arteries or veins, 20 percent result from diabetes, and the remainder are a combination of the above."

On behalf of the American Urological Association, Dr.

Barada led a panel on new treatments in 1996, concluding that oral and topical medications will become the therapies of choice once research efforts are realized. Although Dr. Barada believes there's a place for psychology in treatment, he added, "I've never heard of anybody who's been talked into having an erection."

Thus, using physiologically active substances to deal with impotence works—and there has never been a bigger choice of medications than there is now. The biggest news is the fact that all three of the new types of erectile pills are soon expected to be approved by the FDA, now that medical trials are drawing to a close. Thus, the term "The Pill" has taken on a new meaning in the nineties—and it may lead to another type of sexual revolution.

Thousands of men have already used these pills in the past few years in the United States, Europe, Mexico, and other locations. Some experts say the preliminary results released so far by the drug manufacturers are too optimistic, with erection and satisfaction rates ranging as high as 85 percent. Dr. Barada and others peg the rate at closer to 50 percent. But even if the actual percentage is lower than the 85 percent claimed, it belies the huge amount of satisfaction that many men and their partners gain from these pills. Many were ecstatic.

Fred, a patient in his sixties who lost his ability to have erections due to adult onset diabetes, explained, "The erection pills opened up a whole new world for me again. I felt like I did when I first got married thirty years ago. Due to the diabetes and the medication I've been taking, I became virtually impotent for more than a year. Even when I did get a hard-on and penetrated my wife, it was really unsatisfactory because most of the time I'd end up getting limp. It made me afraid to even try to have intercourse with her because of the fear of being embarrassed if I lost my erection. I was lucky that my urologist got me into a trial group for the new pills. With the pill, I now get an erection and maintain it for a full hour anytime I want to. In fact, it keeps me really hard even after I come so I can keep on going until my wife comes too. She says I'm a real stud again, like I used to be. It makes both of us happy—our marriage has been rejuvenated."

Are the new medications which induce erections true aphrodisiacs? Usually when people refer to aphrodisiacs, there's an implied emphasis placed on the spiritual as well as the physical effects caused by the substance. People want to have a desire to have sex, and they want the ability to enjoy a peak experience while having sex. They also want to fulfil the deepest human urge, that of performing the act of procreation, as well as to enjoy feelings of lust and even love that accompany these close genital penetrations. The new pills and injections will almost certainly enable a man to have an erection and to perform whatever sex acts come to mind—but is the experience satisfying in terms of all the above criteria?

The answer is a resounding *yes*, according to most of the men who have tried them out, as well as their mates. The pills have almost caused a frenzy in some areas—so much so that there was a break-in to steal a batch of the pills at one of the clinics that was conducting trials in San Francisco.

Psychologist Dr. Turkat commented, "Almost invariably, a couple's relationship is improved when they have a satisfactory sexual relationship. For different couples, this can mean anything from having sex once a month, once a week, or twice a day—but whatever a couple chooses to do, the male partner wants to be able to follow through with it. If he needs one of the new medications, so be it—taking them is usually a far better path than not having sex at all, or being nervous about the quality and quantity of sex you have. Sex can help support love, and vice versa."

Urologist Dr. Drogo Montague, director of the Center for Sexual Function at the Cleveland Clinic, reported, "By far, of all the recent developments to treat erectile dysfunction, patients are most excited about the new pills. We're getting requests about these pills nonstop. The concept of being able to simply take a pill when desired and then be virtually assured of having an excellent erection used to be a dream—but now it's a reality. It's a major step forward in our choice of treatments, and it responds to what patients have been hoping for."

In terms of women, Dr. Montague, who also is Professor of Surgery at Ohio State University, added, "Nobody knows the effect that these pills will have on women. I would say that women have been underserved in this field—but I know that men are hoping to have better relationships with women through the use of the new erection medications."

Zonagen, one of the three manufacturers of erectile pills in the United States, has already begun a program to test its product, Vasomax, on women. The basis of the study is the fact that, as with male erectile dysfunction, problems women face with sexual arousal or with reaching orgasm may be associated with vascular circulation. Zonagen is hoping that the active ingredient in Vasomax, phentolamine, will be useful for women as well.

Phentolamine is a vasodilator that acts in about fifteen minutes to relax smooth muscle tissue in the penis and to dilate the arteries—thus leading to an erection in most men who've used it. The majority of these men also ejaculated at least part of the time, while more than forty percent of them ejaculated every single time they had sex. The company is continuing with its studies which it hopes will soon lead to full approval for use in the United States.

The first pill to come on the market was Viagra, made by the giant drug company Pfizer. The active chemical ingredient, sildenafil, has been used in several blinded trials, with up to 92 percent of men reporting they had improved erections. Interestingly, when the same patients received a placebo, only 27 percent reported achieving a satisfactory erection—which goes to prove that sex isn't all in your head. Viagra works by increasing the response to sexual stimulation and increasing blood flow to the penis. The company's literature says, "This may prove to be a dream come true for many patients who are looking for a magic pill to improve their erections." Viagra is meant to be taken an hour before sex. It may cause headache. The active ingredients in Viagra and Vasomax are also being used for successful injection therapy.

The third erectile pill, called Spontane by manufacturer TAP Holdings, works differently from the other two substances. Instead of acting on the physical aspects of erection, it triggers the parts of the brain involved with sex to increase the psychological response to sexual stimulation. In turn, this leads to an erection in up to 70 percent of men. This drug, apomorphine, is best for men with milder cases of erectile dysfunction.

Which pill would be best for you? Even if all three can produce an erection and orgasm, which one will *feel* the best to use? Urologists have no definite answer to this question except to say that all three may have a place in a man's medicine cabinet. San Francisco urologist Dr. Sharlip advises, "It's important for a man to try whatever substance is available to evaluate for himself the effects and satisfaction provided by each of them. At various times in your life you may want to use one, and at other times none at all. If using them, it may be best to alternate the use of substances from time to time for maximum benefit."

One thing is clear, however—the types and availability of aphrodisiacs are growing as never before. And there's bound to be a lot of happy men and women as these aphrodisiacs proliferate.

Ronald, sixty-four, has been a frequent user of the erection pills since he had surgery for prostate cancer two years earlier—and he's thrilled. "Having a pill available when I want to use it seems like a normal part of my life now. I was really depressed after the prostate surgery because I always had enjoyed having sex. It's always been on my mind, ever since I was a teen—so how could I just live without it now? I tried to rationalize it to myself. I'd think, 'Gee Ronald, you only have sex anyway two or three times a week, and it only lasts for maybe twenty minutes, so what's so important about having forty minutes of that particular type of thrill every week? There are hundreds of hours of other enjoyments, including quality time with my girlfriend and grandchildren. And who cares about losing this teeny tiny sexual part of my life when my life has actually been saved by the surgery for cancer? I could have died, but I'm alive!'

"But *damn* it all!" Ronald continued, "Sex really was, is, and always will be an important part of my life. It's hard to pinpoint why. And it's not because I feel like less of a man without it. I have no doubts that I'm a man. It's because I feel like less of a *person* without knowing that I'm a sexual person. Even if I'd only do it once a month or year, I want to know that I *can* do it. The pill I take now works for me.

"My girlfriend, who said she was happy with the way I brought her to orgasm with manual and oral stimulation during the year I was impotent, says she loved me as much during that time as when I was having intercourse with her. But in my heart I feel closer to her spiritually when my penis is inside her and I can see on her face how much she needs that part of me. It's an innate thing, I'm sure.

"I thank God for the new outlook I have on life."

Ronald asked his girlfriend Marilyn, fifty-one, to add a few comments to his experience. She noted, "It's true that I loved Ron before and I love him now. I think the fact that he's so satisfied with his big erections and the fact that he gets to push them into my vagina is what makes me feel stronger toward him. I mean, he's so happy because he's able to please me. Once we were out for a hike in the mountains, and we sat down and ate a couple of sandwiches, and he just casually began caressing my groin and breasts, and I got turned on and surprise, surprise!—I touch him down there and he's got a great big boner. It turns out that he took one of his pills when we got out of the car!

"Well, we were like kids finding a place to hide near some boulders and trees so that the other hikers who were around wouldn't see us. We had sex right there! Ronald certainly didn't need any further foreplay, so we both pulled off our shorts and he casually began screwing me. He was so calm and confident about it, it made it so hot and satisfying for me. He's been very spontaneous about timing our sexual encounters, and that adds to a lot of the fun of it. It's just one more reason for me to love him."

One patient who was given the pills by a Montreal doctor reported that he was in for a big surprise. Alfonso, forty-six, whose frequent impotence stemmed from the fact that he smoked and was overweight, reported, "My doctor had some of the experimental pills in his office, and gave me one right there. He told me to call him as soon as I noticed anything. Jesus—as soon as I got in the elevator something started happening. A pretty dark-haired woman walked in all smelling of perfume. I glanced at her and the frilly lacy underwear thing she had peeking out the top of her blouse, and my cock went boing! I mean, it went straight up in the air, and I practically had to push it down so no one would notice.

"I drove home, and it stayed hard all the way. Luckily, I reached my wife on her cell phone and told her to come home right away because I had a present for her. I got home first, and I lay on our bed naked when she walked in the door—and she just started laughing. She said, 'That's *quite* a present you have there!' and she slid her skirt and panties off, grabbed my erection with her hands, rubbed it around on the outside of her vagina until she got really lubricated, and then sat down on it so I went straight into her. I told her not to rush as she usually did because she'd be scared my hard-on would end too soon. I knew that this erection was going to be around for quite a while. She came and it made her vagina all lubricated and gooey and hot, and she asked me if she could keep on going. I said, 'You do what you want, honey—it all feels great to me'. I came pretty quickly after that, but I stayed hard for another fifteen minutes. My wife and I did a lot of after-play instead of foreplay with making out and stuff like that. It was wonderful. I totally forgot to call the doctor back until the next day—to make sure I could get a good supply of those pills."

A British hospital nurse named Anne, sixty-four explained that she acquired a few of the pills for her husband Charles, sixty-nine. "I was fed up because Charles acted as if he thought that stupid Beatles song 'When I'm 64' was something true—that because I was sixty-four I should be knitting a sweater by the fireside. But I'm a nurse, and I'm in good shape from running around for ten hours a day trying to keep the patients content. Charles was letting me down in the sex department. Whenever I wanted to do it, I had to coax him into it with massages and a shot of port. I got one of the doctors to give me a few of the pills, and I told Charles to take one for his 'vitality' one night when we were going out to dinner. Well his 'vitality' certainly improved. By the time we got back home, he couldn't wait to undress me and make me lick his penis and so on. We had some truly wonderful sex. While he really liked his 'vitality' pills, he began having sex with me more often even when he wasn't taking a pill, because he said the effects lasted for several days. Maybe the extra effect was in his mind, but I'm glad he had something in his mind which involved thinking of me as a sexual partner again."

It's important to note that for all three types of pills, some sexual stimulation is required to actually induce and maintain erections. The stimulation can be provided through physical touch or through a lustful thought going through your mind. Thus, they act as a type of powerful sexual-urge magnifier—like true aphrodisiacs.

### *The Date-rape Pill*

Rohypnol, a very powerful hypontic sedative that can easily render someone unconscious, is absolutely *not* an aphrodisiac.

## The New Pharmacological Substances

It's being included here only to explain that it's highly abusive to use it secretly on women, that it has no place in a respectful sexual relationship, and that it can land you in jail. Rohypnol has been nicknamed "the Date-rape Pill" because guys have been slipping it into the drinks of women they meet at bars or whom they ask on dates—and then these unscrupulous guys have sex with them when they pass out. It's almost a way of simulating necrophilia, or sex with a dead person, because the woman is virtually comatose. This practice seems to appeal to college boys, probably the same ones who daydream of being able to hypnotize women to obey their every command. It seems to be the new "prank" for them to get laid this way—but several are now in jail serving time for this crime.

Police estimate that thousands of girls are victimized by this sleazy tactic each year in the United States, even though only a handful ever lay charges against the perverted perps. "Many girls will wake up and find sperm all over their vaginas or in their anuses or mouths, and realize they've been raped by the guy they went out with. But they're too embarrassed to let everyone know about it, so they never press charges—even though they should," a police spokesperson said.

One woman who did press charges said, "That was a form of violence against me to give me drugs which made me pass out and then to undress me and have sex with me. This guy was a total pervert. In court, he tried to tell the judge that I must have liked it because I didn't object. How could I object if I was unconscious? And the guy's lawyer tried to insinuate that since I was a college girl in a bar with guys that I should expect and accept this kind of crap. I never wanted that guy's penis inside me. Luckily that guy got jail time, and I hope he sits there and rots."

True aphrodisiacs end up making *both* partners happy, so this type of substance should never be confused with one.

### Erection Creams

Creams that you simply rub on your penis to produce an erection are already being tested, but they're not yet available for public use. According to urologist Dr. Sharlip, "If perfected, a localized treatment of this type could become one of the best solutions. Currently, the rub-on preparation contains a form of nitroglycerin and acts as a vasodilator to produce an erection, but it has side effects."

This cream preparation, unfortunately, can bring on a headache in the woman who's at the receiving end of the erection as the drug seeps into her own body. Similarly, if a man uses one of the currently available creams that are designed to prolong erections with a local anesthetic, his woman partner may experience dulled vaginal sensations because of the introduction of the anesthetic into her body by the penis.

It may be a good solution for the man to use a condom once the erection is in force to prevent any passing of the nitroglycerin to his partner, but it remains to be seen if perhaps another chemical works better. Another modality for producing an erection involves increasing the amount of nitric oxide, or NO, within the penis (see page 35). However, the currently available chemicals that encourage the production of NO can't be introduced transdermally as yet—an actual injection into the penis tissue or tip is required. But research is moving forward, fueled on by the potential for huge financial returns.

## Injection Therapy

### ALPROSTADIL, PAPAVERINE, AND PHENTOLAMINE

Although injection treatment is not an aphrodisiac according to the regular definition, it's the forerunner to the development of erection pills for erectile dysfunction, and it's tremendously popular in America. According to urologists, injection therapy will remain popular for at least the next few years simply because it works so well.

There are two methods of introducing any one of the three active chemicals listed above into a man's penis, and both methods are virtually painless. One delivery method involves a thin plastic applicator that shoots the medication in the form of a gel pellet into the tip of the penis. The other method uses a tiny syringe to inject the chemical into the base of the penis. Both delivery methods are readily available through urologists, and both work extremely well—in fact, sometimes too well.

Injection therapy produces a firm erection within five to fifteen minutes, and which lasts for an hour or even two. The wrong dose or combination of drugs, however, can cause a man to acquire a priapism, or permanent erection. This quickly becomes painful—and, if it's not treated within four hours, it can lead to permanent damage of the erectile tissue within the penis. In general, this condition is quite rare for men who are using injection therapy regularly under medical supervision.

Some of the substances used are the same as those found in the erection pills. Combination formulas include alprostadil, papaverine, and phentolamine. A patient can quickly be taught to administer the drugs into his own penis—and they will make virtually any man spring into action in fifteen minutes. While some men feel that it's inconvenient, intrusive, or cumbersome to inject themselves in order to have an erection, injection therapy was a major breakthrough in treatment of erectile dysfunction. It's a sure bet for almost all impotent men, and the ones who've tried it have found this treatment to be a godsend.

But another question arises: Once you acquire this chemically induced erection, do you want to use it? A small group of patients note that while it's true their penises do become as hard as a two-by-four, they don't acquire the urge to have sex with their partner at the same time. "Just because I'm able to stick my hard-on into my wife for as long as I want to, it doesn't make me more turned on to her or to having sex itself," lamented a user named Dino.

Philip, sixty-three, had a practical idea—he takes an herbal aphrodisiac at the same time that he uses injection therapy. "I use the gel applicator now, and it's really excellent. I get an erection that's as stiff and hard as bedrock, and it's really easy to do. And I also found a way to boost my desire for sex at the same time. Prior to starting on this therapy, I had tried a muira puama tea, which was somewhat helpful. Now I'll take it prior to doing the gel application because it makes me feel sexier. My wife sips the tea as well sometimes, and we both end up having excellent orgasms. But she hardly needs any extra stimulation—I can keep on screwing her for as long as she wants because my hard-on stays super-hard for more than an hour. So I can let her get on top of me and move the way she finds most stimulating for herself until she comes. I think we'll be having really good sex for at least another decade."

A twenty-eight-year-old man from Chicago, Brian, reported, "I wanted to impress my girlfriend, so I made an appointment with this urologist who treats my uncle. I kind of lied to him, and told him that I was having trouble getting it up for her because I'm depressed and that she was threatening to leave me. I said if only he could help me screw her a couple of times, I'd be back on the ball. So he got me a prescription for three injections of alprostadil.

"It doesn't hurt at all to use it. A little needle into the cock and that's it. Half an hour later, I was harder than I've ever been in my life. And my cock was super hot and ready to start fucking that little honey pot of my girlfriend Mandy. And she got a real kick out of me! She was fucking me like you wouldn't believe. She kept climaxing and yelling out, 'Oh Brian, oh God, oh Brian.' It's good to know that every once in awhile we can get those stupendous fucks."

As noted, there is some chance of a priapism occurring with injection therapy, and someone who suffers from this must see a doctor immediately. Treatment involves an injection of an antidote or powerful anesthetic into the base of the erection, and may also require a minor surgical procedure to relieve the blood pressure in the penile artery system. Since the chances of this happening are very small, however, and since the other drawbacks are minor, injection therapy will likely remain the treatment of choice for many men for several years.

# 5

# Modern Pharmaceuticals

In the past decade, several new pharmacological substances have emerged in the aphrodisiac field. Two of the best known are L-arginine and niacin, both of which are readily obtainable from drugstores and health food stores. Now that brain activity and brain chemistry are better understood, the psychoactive functions of these substances are being appreciated, as are the newer chemicals on the market.

As noted in chapter 1, deprenyl and bromocriptine were developed to treat the effects of Alzheimer's and Parkinson's—and inadvertently were found to boost the libido as well in both women and men. When these substances are used for sexual purposes, the dosage required is far less than that needed to deal with these major brain problems. Prescriptions are required for these drugs, however, so some conniving may be required if you'd like to try one. As noted earlier, it's legal to get a prescription for so-called off-label use.

## L-arginine

No prescription is needed for L-arginine, which is an essential amino acid. It acts as an aphrodisiac because it increases the body's production of nitric oxide, or NO, in the brain and arteries. This chemical is essential for the production of erections, acting as a type of on-off switch for the penis. Having L-arginine in the bloodstream leads to increased production of NO in the arteries since it gives off nitrogen atoms to combine with blood-born oxygen atoms. The resulting NO molecules seep out of the arteries leading to the penis, relaxing the arterial walls and allowing the penis to become engorged. As the penis enlarges, it constricts the veins that normally allow blood to flow out, producing long-lasting erection. L-arginine also leads to heightened libido and more intense genital-sexual response in women due to its ability to increase blood flow and relax soft muscle tissue. Some women say they start to feel like nymphomaniacs when they're on L-arginine, which is often sold in capsules that also contain Vitamin B-5 and choline.

NO is considered so important now that it was bestowed the title of "Molecule of the Year" by *Science* magazine in 1992 due to its effects in controlling blood pressure, the immune system, cancerous cells, and muscular activity. L-arginine is the primary source of nitrogen molecules needed for the production of NO.

L-arginine became popular in the 1980's among athletes and bodybuilders who took it to boost their performance. That was when the drug was found to boost performance in the bedroom as well as in the stadium. It's considered to be a psychologically mediated aphrodisiac because its actions originate in the brain.

Connie, forty-one, noted that she was quite sexually active in her teens and twenties, and that she enjoyed it. "I had sex with dozens of guys just because I felt like it. But to my surprise I fell in love and got married and stayed faithful for fifteen years. My husband and I had three kids. Unfortunately, he died in a car crash last year. I had completely lost all interest in sex after his death, and I thought I'd never want to make love with any man ever again—and that's what I told this friendly guy next door who was divorced. He suggested I try L-arginine, and I did, and it made me feel like getting laid again. I began screwing around, and I liked it a lot but I didn't want my kids to find out, so I stopped taking the L-arginine and my horniness subsided. But that burst of sex activity got me back into feeling like a woman, so now I'm ready to meet one new man and please the heck out of him. I hope that's enough for me to be happy."

L-arginine tends to make users more aggressive. At first, a German couple, Gitte, forty-two, and Gunther, forty-four, actually appreciated the aggressive attitudes they acquired while using L-arginine for a prolonged period. They said they felt as athletes do when they're on steroids—mean, wild, and wanton. Gitte, said, "We were already heavily using aphrodisiacs with herbs and the occasional hit of Spanish fly, which turned my cunt and my little Liebling's cock into electric fucking machines. The Spanish fly was great, it could keep us going for twenty-four hours of screwing. I'd stick a dildo into Gunther's ass, and he'd stick a giant one in my own ass or pussy, and I'd suck on his cock and slap it and bite it. Man, our orgasms were incredible. But that Spanish fly burned our urethras really a lot, so you can't do it too often.

"Anyway, we started taking a lot of L-arginine at the

health club, and it made our muscles really well-defined. Weight training is great when you're on that. And we began to feel mean.

"I saw Gunther pick a fight with one of our close friends, and I realized we had gone too far and were becoming too crazy from this L-arginine stuff. I think now it's best to take it only once in a while for kicks. That should be enough for anybody."

### *Niacin*

Niacin, also known as vitamin B-3, has a strong aphrodisiac effect on people who enjoy the "flush" they get from it, which is similar to having the entire body blush. This blush comes from the release of histamine in the body, which leads to dilation of blood vessels. The net result is that the body feels very turned on and tingly—as noted years ago by Masters and Johnson. This feeling is often compared to the "sex flush" you may have experienced as you anticipated some wonderful upcoming sex act.

Maureen, twenty-eight, an anthropology student at Cornell, noted, "I appreciate using niacin because it's so fast-acting. It was a surprise to feel that body-blush feeling the first time I tried it, but it does make me feel like I'm perked up and ready for sex and orgasms. The first time I tried it was just after my boyfriend dumped me, and I went to a Halloween costume party in an Ithaca bar with my Cornell girlfriends. I was dressed up as a cat in black tights and a homemade tail. I also had a black mask and whiskers made with an eyebrow pencil. I wanted to be someone different because I was sad about my boyfriend and all that. A guy in a Zorro outfit also had a black mask. He bought me a couple of beers and kept calling me Kitty. He asked me if I wanted to try something different that wasn't pot or coke. We both took the niacin, and I got that overall flushy feeling, like my whole body was blushing—especially my nipples and vagina. They definitely needed to be touched.

"The Zorro guy and I wandered around the bar and found the stairs leading to the empty basement area where they serve the lunch crowd. We began making out in a dark corner. It was really slutty and fun, and I dug it. I kept calling him Zorro, and he kept calling me Kitty. We kept our black masks on the whole time. When he made that first nervous move to put his hand on my breast—like guys do to see if they can get away with it—I put my hand on his hard penis. He almost jumped in surprise. It was obvious his penis was super-sensitive, just like my vagina. I was just really horny from the niacin. The sex took about twenty minutes, and we were back at the party talking with our friends.

"Zorro knew I was a grad student at Cornell, and one day in the classified in our school paper I saw the message 'Zorro desperately seeks Kitty.' I never did call his number. It was great at the time, I was high and horny from that stuff, but since then my boyfriend and I got back together. I bought a bottle of niacin at the pharmacy, and he and I have had really good sex with it too. He wonders how I found out about it, but of course I won't tell him."

### Deprenyl

Deprenyl, an antidepressant, acts in conjunction with the natural brain chemical dopamine to boost the sex drive in most men (and also in older lab animals, who mount and screw like crazy when on this drug). Some researchers believe deprenyl, with the chemical name selegiline hydrochloride, will become known as one of the top ten pharmacological discoveries of the century because of its anti-aging, mind-boosting effects. In fact, several hundred papers have been written about it already, almost all detailing its beneficial effects.

People reported becoming more energetic and having clearer thought patterns. As for animals, United States researchers at Kansas State University said that "youthful vigor" was restored to pet dogs and cats, and that it "reversed symptoms of aging and senility." These older pets became much more alert when they were on deprenyl—for instance, dogs wouldn't urinate indoors and wouldn't wander aimlessly as they used to. In fact, the researchers concluded that animals would live years longer if they were given deprenyl in their food. This has led to the medical opinion that people too will live longer if they take deprenyl.

To top off all of this, both humans and animals became hornier and more sexually active when on it. A doctor noted, "Not only are these older fellows gaining relief from depression and becoming mentally sharper, they're also getting better at screwing their spouses."

Regarding younger people, many who had been taking Prozac for depression were switched to deprenyl by their physicians because the Prozac was interfering with their ability to have orgasms. These young men and women were also surprised to find their sex drives and orgasm frequency were greatly boosted.

Both the older and younger people are known to be sharing their pills with friends. A woman named Brynn, thirty-six, said, "On Prozac, I'd end up having intercourse with my boyfriend for half an hour, but I'd never have an orgasm. Before I started on it, I'd come within a normal time span of about five minutes. The frustrating part is that I'd be *wanting*, even *yearning* to come as the base of his penis hit my vulva and clitoris over and over. I'd be begging for my body to release itself in an orgasm, but it wouldn't happen. I practically cried from the disappointment each time. My doctor advised me to take Prozac vacations for a weekend, and I might have an orgasm if I was lucky on Sunday—but that was no solution.

"When my doctor got me to try deprenyl, everything went so well that my boyfriend insisted on trying it too. He saw that I was in a good mood and that my orgasms were very pleasurable, so he took a little bit of a day's worth. We ended up screwing like crazy for a whole week. His manhood had so much get-up-and-go that it hardly went down at all. And I had multiple orgasms until my vagina hurt from all the friction. I think that week we made up for a whole year of lousy sex."

Tyler, thirty-two, reported, "I took some of the pills from my dad's medicine cabinet because I heard him talking to his friend about how good it was. He was bragging that he was able to pork my mom almost every night because he was getting so many boners. Well, it sure worked on me too. My girlfriend Ginny likes spontaneous sex, and so do I, but I get nervous and don't always have a hard-on in these strange locations she picks, like bathrooms, changing rooms, cars, and closets. I started getting so many boners right after trying those stolen pills that I was finally able to be her match. I was able to screw her anywhere I was close enough to press my cock into her cunt.

"The more difficult it is to twist our bodies the right way around to be able to get our sex organs together, the more erotic it is for us. I have a sports car with a stick shift, so when we do it in the car I usually move onto Ginny's seat while she straddles me. She digs it because she gets to control the whole thing by being on top."

Howard, sixty-five, was legitimately prescribed deprenyl for a mental condition. "I was in a lethargic frame of mind and body for a year before I sought help from my physician. I hadn't had intercourse with my wife for all that time, and I didn't even feel bad about it for her sake or miss it myself. I just didn't care. Once I was on deprenyl, I became more energetic, and I did begin to have feelings and interests again. My wife was as surprised as I was when I began doing foreplay with her. I had almost forgotten how! I reached over to her in our bed after we had come back from a night of bridge, and I began caressing her breasts and then her vagina. She said, 'I thought you'd never touch me in that way again,' and it made me feel sad. I was grateful that I was able to have really nice sex with her, that I'm able to be a husband to her again. We do it now about once a week, and we're much happier with each other."

### *Bromocriptine*

Bromocriptine can work as an aphrodisiac in both younger and older people, whether or not they're having any sexual dysfunction. In older men and women, it helps bring sexual activity up to higher levels even in cases of male impotence, mainly by countering the normal effects of aging on our pituitary glands. As we get older, these glands produce more prolactin, which becomes too much of a good thing. Excess prolactin is linked with erectile and orgasmic dysfunction—

and the prescription drug bromocriptine brings prolactin levels down to normal levels in almost everyone who takes it.

Another bonus of bromocriptine is that it stimulates production of dopamine and is a mild antidepressant. Because it affects brain activity, it can make people desire sex more and give orgasms a kick start.

Allan, seventy-five, said that he was happy that his *desire* for sex went up along with his ability to have sex once he started a course of bromocriptine. "A couple of years ago, I began having fewer thoughts and daydreams about sex. I became very despondent because it seemed like a part of me, my sexual being, was gone. I almost never had intercourse with my wife, and I was usually only able to bring her to orgasm manually.

"I knew I was getting older, but I heard that guys as old as Abraham were able to have sex and even babies, so why not me? I always liked sex, even if I had less of it as the years went by. I was determined to see if I could fix my problem. After much research and talking to doctors and friends, I simply tried taking bromocriptine and the results were really fine. I began to want sex again and to have the confidence that I would be able to do it satisfactorily again. My wife Mona is only sixty-five, so she was very pleased when I told her I seemed to be getting ready for action again."

Allen continued, "We were out for a morning walk on the boardwalk in North Miami, and for a lark we strolled down near the nudist section at Haulover Beach. It was kind of fun seeing all the nudists playing volleyball and lounging around in the buff. Mona got a kick out of seeing all the penises flipping up in the air as the players jumped at the volleyball nets. There certainly was every type of body shape imaginable, and my imagination was working overtime. We went back to our condo for a shower, and when she came out I took her by the hand to our bed and my feelings were accurate—my penis developed into an excellent erection and I screwed her as if I was thirty years younger. We both had really good orgasms, and I've been able to have my way with her a couple of times a week since then. And I'm back to thinking about having sex much more often than that."

Another couple, Jacqueline and Ernest, married for ten years and now in their late sixties, were having decent sex in terms of penetration, but both were missing out on having orgasms about half the time. Ernest said, "We'd be screwing away for five or ten minutes and then my hard-on would start to go down. I'd want to shoot my wad off into Jacqueline, but it wouldn't happen. And on the times when my cock did work perfectly, she might not have an orgasm even if she played with her own clitoris while I fucked her.

"Jacqueline's bridge partner advised her that both of us should get on bromocriptine, and it's made a huge difference. We take it for a few weeks from time to time, and we both have great orgasms again. We're having intercourse all the time, and we dig it. I'm looking forward to having nice sex with her until the day we die."

A sixty-one-year-old therapist, Lorna, began seeing a forty-year-old man with strange tastes. Lorna noted, "Jim, my new man, likes it when I tie him up to a narrow weight-lifting bench with his belt and then rub mentholated sore-muscle cream on his penis. He gets hard as a rock. Then I'm supposed to straddle his face and order him to lick my vagina—and then I'm supposed to mount him and screw him until he comes. Don't forget, he can't move because of the leather straps. I do it because we love each other, but I hadn't been feeling all that energetic sexually. All of his demands placed a big onus on me, obviously. So one of my colleagues prescribed bromocriptine for me and I began feeling far more sexual. My vagina feels more perky and gets itself primed for orgasms much better than before—so that makes me better at screwing him while he lies tied down that way. He comes and I come, and we're both happy. That's what love is all about."

Two important points to note about bromocriptine are that it may produce too much clitoral stimulation, bringing on a temporary painful condition of clitoral tumescence. It may also bring on ovulation and hence pregnancy in women who are at or near menopause.

People reading about the effects of deprenyl and other substances described in this book may wonder, will this work for me? Well, as we've been saying, why not just try it and see? The low dosages required for aphrodisiac effects produce few harmful side effects, so what's there to lose? Certain combinations of substances are to be avoided, such as deprenyl with yohimbine, and you can find this out along with the proper doses from a knowledgeable physician. Some substances work extremely well on some people and some don't. As noted, it's important to find out what's good for your body type—and, it's a great excuse to ask someone to have sex with you!

# 6

# The Aphrodisiac Feast

Where else to go but the City of Love, San Francisco, to find the best in food aphrodisiacs?

Perhaps the finest aphrodisiac food feast in the country is offered at the Millennium restaurant at the base of the historic Abigail Hotel on McAllister street. Once a month, on the Sunday falling closest to the full moon, the Millennium offers Aphrodisiac Night, a very sensual and popular five-course vegetarian aphrodisiac feast that includes a now-infamous love potion invented by legendary herbalist Dr. Tom Dunphy. An alluring feature of Aphrodisiac Nights is that a night in the ornate hotel is provided as part of the all-inclusive dinner menu.

The feast is always sold out weeks in advance. With the right planning, though, you can always stage an aphrodisiac feast of your own if you can't make it to San Francisco at the right time.

Randall Reeves, the Millennium's general manager, explained, "Our chef did a lot of research into aphrodisiac foods and dishes, and we put in a lot of effort in purchasing the finest seasonal ingredients. We also have a lovely atmosphere, but the dishes can be prepared by anyone with the right touch. For couples who want it all done for them, we've become a very popular attraction, and many interesting things happen on those special nights. We wouldn't consider sending couples away into the night after the sensuousness of a dinner like that, so we provide hotel accommodations for every couple. In fact, many couples have become engaged over dinner before heading to their rooms. Guys actually pull out diamond rings right at the tables. Men and women bring in lots of flowers, especially roses, which we place on their tables. Our biggest night is Valentine's, and we could sell ten times as many places as we have available. And the morning after each feast, the hotel lobby is full of people walking around with big smiles."

Alice, a woman who's been on the scene, noted wistfully, "All kinds of things go on during Aphrodisiac Nights. There's lots of touching and smooching, caressing of hair and arms, lots of eye contact, loving looks, and warm hand holding. It's very beautiful. I've heard there were times when singles showed up and ended up pairing off as they headed toward the upstairs hotel rooms. I wanted to be one of them."

Reeves pointed out that the popularity of the monthly event has spread throughout San Francisco simply by word of mouth. "We started Aphrodisiac Nights in 1995, and it was an instant success. When the right foods are prepared in a luxurious way, the aphrodisiac qualities affect everybody. Our menu features exotic foods, herbs, spices, and wild mushrooms prepared by our specially trained chef. Our clients are very enthusiastic about these romantic and sexy dishes, and we get a lot of repeat business. Clients range in age from their late twenties to their fifties and sixties. Some admit that an extra bonus for their sensual evening is the fact that they're escaping from their children for the night.

"In between courses, couples have the option of taking a sojourn up to their room for an hour or so if they desire, and many do pick up their wineglasses and head discreetly upstairs for awhile. It's nice to see people holding hands and putting their arms around each other and just carrying on like young lovers."

The chef, Eric Tucker, who outlined many of his excellent aphrodisiac recipes in his recent book, *The Millennium Cookbook,* explained, "For centuries it's been known that certain foods cooked in just the right way are good for love and the libido. We've done a lot of research with herbalists and gourmet chefs to come up with the best combination of foods for an aphrodisiac night. The most active ingredients I use are the herb damiana, which goes into the salad dressing; ginseng, which I typically lace through curried vegetables; saffron; and, exotic mushrooms. If we weren't a vegetarian restaurant, I'd add shellfish such as oysters, mussels, and shrimp."

Chef Tucker added, "Our typical menu includes a jasmine rice-shitake salad with a damiana dressing; smoked tofu; avocado and cilantro; crisp pastry filled with marinated seitan, oyster mushrooms, and basil, served over a ginseng-curry sauce; basil fettucine sautéed in a wild mushroom-saffron sauce with Jerusalem artichokes; and a warm pudding cake served over coconut cardamom sauce. The exotic mushrooms are especially important because they're known to stimulate the erotic zones.

"For starters, we begin with pickled things such as olives, capers, and other vegetables. When available, we include items such as hijiki or arame seaweed, matzutake or lobster mushrooms, artichoke since it's a member of the thistle family, and a basil/pomegranate sauce. For dessert, we'll usually have a chocolate-based dish that's either savory or sweet—for instance a molee or a mousse. And there'll be tropical fruits such as mangoes and strawberries.

"Each item is planned to stroke all the senses and to build upon each other in a sensual progression. And there are aphrodisiacs and nutrients within the food, all of which is designed to give you a healthful, fresh feeling. While we never serve meat anyway, it's not considered to have aphrodisiac qualities, so I wouldn't include meat dishes in this type of dinner. Of course, we always serve Dr. Dunphy's famous Love Potion Number Nine with dinner, and that adds to the overall amazing effect that our dinner provides."

Love Potion Number Nine is a very special aphrodisiac invented by the legendary Dr. Dunphy, a pharmacist, herbalist, and acupuncturist who founded the Herbal Apothecary in San Francisco. Although Dr. Dunphy has crossed over to the other side and didn't answer our request for an interview, his unique Love Potion continues to fascinate and stimulate amorous couples. It's made from the essences of a combination of nine exotic herbs specially formulated to react with each other to produce the maximum aphrodisiac effects. A dropperful of Love Potion Number Nine is all that's needed for a night of love, according to those who've tried it at the Millennium.

While it would be extremely difficult for anyone to reproduce Love Potion Number Nine, the current owners of the Herbal Apothecary have graciously agreed to list the nine ingredients of the late Dr. Dunphy's amazing potion for readers of this book. Here, published for the first time, are the nine ingredients for Love Potion Number Nine: ginseng, rehmannia, cornus, hoelen, dioscorea, moutan, alisma, aconite, and cinnamon.

Reeves said that after the Love Potion Number Nine is delivered to his restaurant, it's prepared for Aphrodisic Night guests by stirring a dropperful into a mixture of pomegranate juice with a dash of lemon and lime, and pouring it into a martini glass. "Everyone who's tried this tonic is very keen to have it again. Some have said they've had beautiful, amorous experiences after trying the potion. It really turns people on."

A couple who's enjoyed the Millennium restaurant reported that the best part of their dining experience was the fact that their excitement kept mounting higher and higher during the dinner. Maggie, who's forty-five, said, "By the time we lay down on our bed a few flights up, we were really, really ready to make love. Our mouths, lips, and tongues had become so sensitized by all the amazing flavors and textures that my husband and I simply tore off each other's clothes and began licking every part of each other's bodies. He tasted so *good* to me. I'm sure my love level for him went up along with my libido level. Both of us also felt so healthy, as if our cardiovascular system was energized by the aphrodisiacs in the food and that Love Potion they give you.

"We began having sex with all the lights on, marveling at how beautiful we both looked in our sexual union. My vagina felt like a warm, open, mushy flower just waiting to receive my husband's very manly and hard cock. I loved receiving his erection into me that night. We were both pretty close to climaxing right away, but we moved slowly and prolonged it for as long as we could, then had wonderful gushy orgasms and napped for an hour. When we woke up, we still felt energized, so we had a warm, leisurely bubble bath in a flowery-scented lotion provided by the hotel, finished off a martini glass full of the pomegranate and Love Potion cocktail we had brought upstairs earlier, and went back to bed and started all over again."

Maggie added, "This time I got on top because my husband wanted to lie back and enjoy the love. His penis stood up straight like the Eiffel Tower, and I licked it and teased him with my mouth, lips, and tongue. He went slightly crazy, which was the general idea. I straddled his face and let him lick my vulva as I rocked back and forth over his mouth while I reached back and caressed his Eiffel Tower of a cock. I told him he felt like he was nineteen years old in my hands! I slid my pussy back down to his groin and began fucking him like I was riding a horse. My vagina and clit were going wild, and those sensational sexual vibes were making me shudder with pleasure. He squeezed and caressed my breasts, and man, when we came again, it was wild. It made me remember why we got married in the first place fifteen years ago. He promised to take me back to the Millennium for my birthday in a few months, and that'll be a treat to remember."

Maggie added, "One funny thought that crossed my mind was the fact that our two kids would never believe what a pair of hot and horny people their parents are. Some things are best kept secret! (And please don't put our real names in your book!)"

Another couple said it was really funny to watch the other Aphrodisiac Night guests. "The couples are spread out in the restaurant mostly with only one couple at a table—but there were a few tables with three and four people at them. You could see people looking at each other and catching each other's eyes even from across the room as their sexual-readiness levels built up with the various courses. Even the threesomes and foursomes would all be touching each other discreetly, rubbing their shoulders together and stroking each other's arms, and talking animatedly.

"I walked by one of the rooms later when a bellhop was delivering some wine, and I caught a peek through the open door. There were strange goings-on with people dressed in leather outfits. The whole hotel seemed to be buzzing with sexuality."

# 7

# Miscellaneous Aphrodisiac Information

### Animal Products

Many animal-based products that have a tradition of being aphrodisiacs are illegal, and this seems to give them a mystical aura. Interestingly, many Asian herbalists say that these products boost the power of a man's sperm rather than that of his erection—so they're not actually in the category of aphrodisiacs even to these experts. Prized animal products include gallstones, bear gallbladders, raw or living monkey brain, rhino horn, and the penises and testicles of tigers, seals, lions, wolves, deer, and even crocodile. The idea is that the part of the animal that you admire while it's alive (usually the penis) will give you similar powers in that same part of your body if you eat it or make a tea out of it. Along the same lines, it was thought in the past that vegetables that were in the shape of genitals had aphrodisiac properties. Thus carrots, celery, and asparagus were prized, as were avocados because they resemble the scrotum.

These animal parts have been subjected to in-depth analysis in the United States, with results indicating that you're not missing much if you pass them by. Professor Corrie Brown, head of the Department of Veterinary Pathology at the University of Georgia, explained, "The meat making up the penises of these animals doesn't yield any physiologically active substances that are different from the meat found in other parts of the animal. Even if there would be any substances such as testosterone present, cooking these items in a soup or tea as is often done would totally leach out any possible hormonal activity. Also, items like rhinoceros horn are made up almost totally of keratin, the same substance found in abundance in our own hair, nails, and skin. There's no reason why ingesting more of this keratin from rhino horns or rhino toenails would have any effect of any type on the libido."

In terms of renewable animal products, the furry covering shed from deer antlers is always available in Asian herbal shops, as is bird spittle found in the nests of sea swallows.

Interestingly, I received hardly any feedback from people regarding successful use of any of these animal products while preparing this book. And, many men have been ripped off—spending $650 for "seal" penises—which turned out to be dried dog penises!

In talking about illegal substances, a gentleman who lived in China before it turned communist noted that he went to an opium den and had such a wild sexual weekend that he remembers all the details even fifty years later. Alfred said, "I just couldn't stop having sex for an entire weekend with woman after woman. I must have had intercourse with about a dozen different women. Some were prostitutes and some were women I picked up at the local dance halls. It was the most amazing and fascinating experience. I remember having all these naked, beautiful women in between my legs and receiving pure pleasure from them. The wonderful feeling of flesh on flesh. I felt really alive. It was sex, sex, and more sex. I couldn't get enough. I couldn't stop. I felt like a superman. I often think of those few days and how exciting it would be to do it all over again. It was one of the highlights of my life. But I got married, moved to Canada, and tried to put it all out of my mind. If ever there was an aphrodisiac worth using, it's opium."

## Spanish Fly

One so-called aphrodisiac that everyone in the world seems to have heard of and that everyone should also avoid is Spanish fly. Physicians are unanimous in stating that this substance, made from ground-up parts of the Cantharis beetle, may be harmful. Rather than making a person actually feel sexually aroused, it acts by irritating the urinary tract, including the bladder and genitals—providing a fake sexual "itch." The itch can go on long after sex and it can drive you crazy. For some people, moreover, ingesting these insect parts can be fatal. So stay away from this one!

## Vacuum Devices and Penile Implants

It's true that you really can put a little round tube around your penis and use it to give you an erection. As the idea implies, a man places his penis into the tube, and pumps a little squeegee ball a few times to create a vacuum in the tube, causing his penis to become erect. Then a kind of rubber band is rolled to the base of the penis, the tube is removed, and voila—the man has an erection for as long as the band is left in place. While it's a cumbersome procedure, it usually works and men do have orgasms.

Penile implants are a far more serious matter, requiring surgery and up to three weeks for full recovery. A small device is placed into the penis permanently, and when it's activated through a control embedded in the area of the groin, it makes the penis rigid.

Anyone considering these choices can get all the details, benefits, and drawbacks from a urologist. Usually these are done as a last resort, but they're a real benefit for the right patient.

### Mixing and Matching

It's important to note that you can usually mix aphrodisiacs together for a stronger effect. In general, there's no reason not to mix and match the various herbs to find the combinations that work best for you. There are some counterindications, however, when you're taking the pharmaceuticals. For instance, deprenyl and yohimbine shouldn't be taken together. A health professional can guide you in finding safe and effective combinations.

During the course of a particular weekend, you may enjoy trying one category of substances, and then switching to another category for your next sexual excursion. As we noted previously, different people prefer different combinations. Experimentation is the key to satisfaction.

# Selected Bibliography

Allardice, Pamela: *Aphrodisiacs and Love Magic,* Avery Publishing Group, 1989
Ishihara, Akira and Levy, Howard S.: *The Tao of Sex,* Paragon Book Gallery, 1986
Lee, Vera, Ph.D.: *Secrets of Venus,* Mt. Ivy Press, 1996
Miller, Richard Alan: *The Magical and Ritual Use of Aphrodisiacs,* Destiny Books, 1985, 1993
Morganthaler, John and Joy, Dan: *Better Sex Through Chemistry.* Smart Publications, 1994
The Treatment of Organic Erectile Dysfunction, The American Urological Association Erectile Dysfunction Clinical Guidelines Panel, 1996
Warburton, Diana: *A-Z of Aphrodisia,* HarperCollins, 1986, 1995
Watson, Cynthia M., M.D. and Hynes, Angela: *Love Potions,* Putnam, 1993
Wedeck, H. E.: *Dictionary of Aphrodisiacs,* Bracken Books, 1962, 1994